# THE DR. BARBARA

# DIABETES COOKBOOK FOR BEGINNERS

365 Days Easy to prepare Mouthwatering Recipes for Diabetes Type 1 and Type 2 inspired by the dr barbara lost cookbook to Combat the Effects of Processed Foods + 28-Days Meal Plan

Rachel Castro

# A Note to My Readers

Dear Readers,

Thank you for choosing "**THE DR. BARBARA O'NEILL DIABETES COOKBOOK FOR BEGINNERS**." I hope you find this book as insightful and helpful as I intended it to be. Your journey to better health is important to me, and I would love to hear about your experiences with the book.

If you found the recipes, herbal remedies, and meal plans beneficial, or if you have any suggestions for improvement, I kindly ask you to share your thoughts through an honest review on Amazon. Your feedback is invaluable and will help me refine future editions to better serve you and others on the path to managing and reversing diabetes naturally.

Thank you for your support and for taking the time to provide your honest review. Your insights mean the world to me and to future readers.

Warm regards,

Rachel Castro

# Introduction

Welcome to **THE DR. BARBARA O'NEILL DIABETES COOKBOOK FOR BEGINNERS**, a comprehensive guide designed to help you reverse diabetes naturally through delicious recipes, herbal remedies, and a 28-day meal plan. Whether you have been recently diagnosed with type 1 or type 2 diabetes, or you have been living with the condition for years, this book offers a transformative approach to managing and potentially reversing your diabetes.

## The Power of Nutrition and Herbal Remedies

Diabetes can feel like an overwhelming and insurmountable challenge. The constant monitoring of blood sugar levels, the endless medications, and the dietary restrictions can take a toll on both your physical and mental health. But what if there was a way to take control of your health and reduce your dependence on medications? Dr. Barbara O'Neill's approach combines the healing power of nutrition with herbal remedies to offer a natural and effective way to manage diabetes.

Dr. Barbara O'Neill, a renowned expert in natural health, has dedicated her life to helping individuals achieve optimal health through natural means. Her methods focus on harnessing the power of whole foods and medicinal herbs to stabilize blood sugar levels and improve overall health. This cookbook is a culmination of her years of research and practical experience, offering you the tools you need to embark on a journey towards better health.

## What You'll Discover in This Book

In **THE DR. BARBARA O'NEILL DIABETES COOKBOOK FOR BEGINNERS**, you will find a wealth of information and practical guidance to help you manage and potentially reverse diabetes. Here's a glimpse of what awaits you:

**Understanding Diabetes:** Gain a clear understanding of what diabetes is, its causes, symptoms, and the impact it has on your health

**The Role of Diet:** Learn about the critical role that nutrition plays in managing diabetes, including the importance of balancing macronutrients and understanding the glycemic index.

**Herbal Remedies:** Discover the healing properties of essential herbs such as bitter melon, fenugreek, and cinnamon, and learn how to incorporate them into your daily routine safely and effectively.

**28-Day Meal Plan:** Follow a structured, easy-to-follow meal plan that takes the guesswork out of planning your meals. This plan includes delicious recipes for breakfast, lunch, dinner, and snacks, all designed to help stabilize your blood sugar levels.

**365 Days of Mouthwatering Recipes:** Enjoy a variety of recipes that are not only diabetes-friendly but also incredibly tasty. From breakfast smoothies to hearty dinners and guilt-free desserts, you'll find something to satisfy every craving.

**Lifestyle Changes:** Understand the importance of lifestyle changes such as regular exercise and stress management, and learn how to incorporate these practices into your daily life.

**Success Stories and Testimonials:** Be inspired by real-life stories of individuals who have successfully managed or even reversed their diabetes using Dr. Barbara's methods. These stories provide hope and motivation, proving that change is possible.

## Your Journey to Better Health Starts Here

This book is more than just a cookbook; it's a roadmap to better health. By following the guidance and recipes in this book, you can take control of your diabetes and transform your life. Imagine waking up each day with more energy, improved health, and the knowledge that you are doing everything you can to manage your diabetes naturally.

As you embark on this journey, remember that you are not alone. Dr. Barbara O'Neill's approach has helped countless individuals achieve better health, and it can help you too. The path to reversing diabetes is not always easy, but with commitment and the right tools, it is entirely possible.

## Let's Get Started

So, are you ready to take control of your health? Are you ready to embrace a new way of eating that nourishes your body and supports your journey to reversing diabetes? If so, then let's get started. Open this book, explore the wealth of knowledge within its pages, and begin your journey to a healthier, happier you.

Welcome to **THE DR. BARBARA O'NEILL DIABETES COOKBOOK FOR BEGINNERS**, your guide to reversing diabetes naturally, one delicious recipe at a time.

# Chapter 1: Understanding Diabetes

## 1.1 What is Diabetes?

Diabetes is a chronic metabolic disorder characterized by high levels of glucose (sugar) in the blood. This condition arises either due to the body's inability to produce enough insulin or because the body cannot effectively use the insulin it produces. Insulin, a hormone produced by the pancreas, plays a crucial role in regulating blood sugar levels by facilitating the uptake of glucose into cells, where it is used for energy. When insulin function is impaired, glucose accumulates in the bloodstream, leading to hyperglycemia.

### Types of Diabetes

There are three main types of diabetes: Type 1, Type 2, and Gestational Diabetes.

### Type 1 Diabetes

Type 1 diabetes, also known as insulin-dependent diabetes or juvenile diabetes, is an autoimmune condition where the body's immune system attacks and destroys the insulin-producing beta cells in the pancreas. This results in little to no insulin production. People with Type 1 diabetes require lifelong insulin therapy to manage their blood glucose levels. This type of diabetes often develops in childhood or adolescence, but it can occur at any age.

## Type 2 Diabetes

Type 2 diabetes is the most common form of diabetes, accounting for about 90-95% of all diabetes cases. It is often referred to as adult-onset diabetes, although it is increasingly diagnosed in children and adolescents due to rising obesity rates. In Type 2 diabetes, the body becomes resistant to insulin, and the pancreas is unable to produce sufficient insulin to overcome this resistance. Lifestyle factors such as obesity, physical inactivity, and poor diet significantly contribute to the development of Type 2 diabetes.

## Gestational Diabetes

Gestational diabetes occurs during pregnancy and usually resolves after childbirth. It is diagnosed when higher-than-normal blood glucose levels are detected in a pregnant woman who did not have diabetes before pregnancy. Although gestational diabetes is temporary, it increases the risk of developing Type 2 diabetes later in life for both the mother and the child.

## Causes and Risk Factors

The exact cause of diabetes varies depending on the type. However, several common factors contribute to the development of the disease.

## Genetic Factors

Genetics play a significant role in both Type 1 and Type 2 diabetes. A family history of diabetes increases the risk of developing the condition. Specific genetic mutations can also predispose individuals to diabetes by affecting insulin production or action.

## Environmental Factors

Environmental factors, such as viral infections, may trigger the onset of Type 1 diabetes in genetically susceptible individuals. For Type 2 diabetes, lifestyle factors are critical. A sedentary lifestyle, poor diet, and obesity are major risk factors. Additionally, aging increases the risk of Type 2 diabetes as the body's ability to process glucose declines over time.

## Other Risk Factors

Other risk factors for diabetes include:

Ethnicity: Certain ethnic groups, such as African Americans, Hispanics, Native Americans, and Asians, have a higher risk of developing diabetes.

History of Gestational Diabetes: Women who have had gestational diabetes are at higher risk for developing Type 2 diabetes later in life.

Polycystic Ovary Syndrome (PCOS): Women with PCOS are at increased risk for Type 2 diabetes.

Hypertension and Hyperlipidemia: High blood pressure and high cholesterol levels are associated with an increased risk of Type 2 diabetes.

## Symptoms and Diagnosis

The symptoms of diabetes can vary depending on the type and severity of the condition. Common symptoms include:

Increased Thirst and Urination: High blood glucose levels cause excess glucose to be excreted in the urine, leading to increased urination and thirst.

Extreme Hunger: Despite eating, people with diabetes may feel excessively hungry because their cells are not receiving enough glucose.

Unintended Weight Loss: The body may start breaking down fat and muscle for energy due to the inability to use glucose effectively, leading to weight loss.

Fatigue: Lack of glucose in cells can result in tiredness and fatigue.

Blurred Vision: High blood sugar levels can cause fluid to be pulled from the lenses of the eyes, affecting vision.

Slow-Healing Sores or Frequent Infections: Poor circulation and immune function can slow the healing process and increase the risk of infections.

## Diagnosis of Diabetes

Diabetes is diagnosed through several tests that measure blood glucose levels:

Fasting Plasma Glucose (FPG) Test: This test measures blood glucose after an overnight fast. A fasting blood sugar level of 126 mg/dL (7.0 mmol/L) or higher on two separate occasions indicates diabetes.

Oral Glucose Tolerance Test (OGTT): This test involves fasting overnight, drinking a sugary solution, and measuring blood glucose levels two hours later. A blood sugar level of 200 mg/dL (11.1 mmol/L) or higher indicates diabetes.

Glycated Hemoglobin (A1C) Test: This test provides an average blood sugar level over the past two to three months. An A1C level of 6.5% or higher on two separate occasions indicates diabetes.

Random Plasma Glucose Test: A blood sugar level of 200 mg/dL (11.1 mmol/L) or higher at any time, regardless of when you last ate, combined with symptoms of diabetes, indicates diabetes.

# 1.2: The Impact of Diabetes on Health

Diabetes is a chronic condition that affects millions of people worldwide. Its impact on health can be profound and multifaceted, affecting nearly every system in the body. Understanding the potential complications and health risks associated with diabetes is crucial for both preventing the disease and managing it effectively once diagnosed. In this section, we will explore the short-term and long-term complications of diabetes, as well as the importance of early detection and management in mitigating these risks.

## Short-term Complications of Diabetes

### Hypoglycemia (Low Blood Sugar):

Definition and Causes: Hypoglycemia occurs when blood sugar levels drop below the normal range, typically due to excessive insulin or certain diabetes medications, skipping meals, or intense physical activity.

Symptoms: Common symptoms include shakiness, sweating, dizziness, confusion, irritability, and in severe cases, loss of consciousness or seizures.

Management: Immediate consumption of fast-acting carbohydrates, such as glucose tablets, juice, or candy, can quickly raise blood sugar levels. Regular monitoring and adjustments to medication and diet are essential to prevent recurrence.

## Hyperglycemia (High Blood Sugar):

Definition and Causes: Hyperglycemia occurs when blood sugar levels are excessively high, often due to insufficient insulin, overeating, stress, or illness.

Symptoms: Symptoms include frequent urination, excessive thirst, blurred vision, fatigue, and headaches. Severe hyperglycemia can lead to diabetic ketoacidosis (DKA) or hyperosmolar hyperglycemic state (HHS), both of which are medical emergencies.

Management: Treatment involves adjusting medications, staying hydrated, and monitoring blood sugar levels closely. In severe cases, hospitalization may be required.

## Diabetic Ketoacidosis (DKA):

Definition and Causes: DKA is a life-threatening condition that occurs when the body breaks down fat for energy in the absence of sufficient insulin, leading to the production of ketones, which accumulate in the blood and cause acidosis.

Symptoms: Symptoms include nausea, vomiting, abdominal pain, rapid breathing, fruity-scented breath, and confusion.

Management: Immediate medical attention is required, with treatment involving insulin therapy, fluid replacement, and electrolyte management.

## Hyperosmolar Hyperglycemic State (HHS):

Definition and Causes: HHS is a serious condition characterized by extremely high blood sugar levels without the presence of ketones. It is more common in older adults with type 2 diabetes.

Symptoms: Symptoms include extreme thirst, frequent urination, dry skin, fever, drowsiness, and altered mental status.

Management: Similar to DKA, HHS requires emergency medical care, including fluid replacement, insulin therapy, and correction of electrolyte imbalances.

# Long-term Complications of Diabetes

## Cardiovascular Disease:

Definition and Causes: People with diabetes are at a significantly higher risk of developing cardiovascular diseases, including coronary artery disease, heart attack, and stroke. This is due to the damaging effects of high blood sugar on blood vessels and the presence of additional risk factors such as hypertension and dyslipidemia.

Management: Managing blood sugar levels, blood pressure, and cholesterol through medication, diet, and lifestyle changes can reduce the risk of cardiovascular complications. Regular physical activity and smoking cessation are also crucial.

## Neuropathy (Nerve Damage):

Definition and Causes: Chronic high blood sugar can damage nerves throughout the body, leading to diabetic neuropathy. Peripheral neuropathy affects the extremities, while autonomic neuropathy affects internal organs.

Symptoms: Peripheral neuropathy symptoms include pain, tingling, numbness, and loss of sensation in the hands and feet. Autonomic neuropathy can cause digestive issues, bladder problems, sexual dysfunction, and cardiovascular abnormalities.

Management: Good blood sugar control, pain management, and proper foot care are essential in managing neuropathy. Medications and therapies can also help alleviate symptoms.

## Nephropathy (Kidney Damage):

Definition and Causes: Diabetic nephropathy is a leading cause of chronic kidney disease (CKD) and end-stage renal disease (ESRD). High blood sugar levels damage the kidneys' filtering system, leading to protein leakage and reduced kidney function.

Symptoms: Early stages may have no symptoms, but as the condition progresses, symptoms such as swelling, fatigue, and high blood pressure may appear.

Management: Controlling blood sugar and blood pressure, along with regular kidney function monitoring, can slow the progression of nephropathy. In advanced stages, dialysis or kidney transplantation may be necessary.

## Retinopathy (Eye Damage):

Definition and Causes: Diabetic retinopathy is a common complication where high blood sugar damages the blood vessels in the retina, potentially leading to vision loss and blindness.

Symptoms: Early stages may be asymptomatic. As the condition progresses, symptoms can include blurry vision, floaters, dark or empty areas in the vision, and difficulty seeing at night.

Management: Regular eye exams, good blood sugar control, and treatments such as laser therapy or injections can help manage retinopathy and prevent vision loss.

## Foot Complications:

Definition and Causes: Diabetes can lead to various foot problems, including infections, ulcers, and, in severe cases, amputations. Poor circulation and neuropathy increase the risk of foot complications.

Symptoms: Symptoms include pain, sores, infections, and changes in skin color or temperature.

Management: Proper foot care, regular inspections, and early treatment of any issues are critical. Wearing appropriate footwear and managing blood sugar levels can help prevent complications.

## Skin Complications:

Definition and Causes: Diabetes can make the skin more susceptible to bacterial and fungal infections, as well as other conditions such as diabetic dermopathy and necrobiosis lipoidica.

Symptoms: Symptoms vary depending on the condition but can include rashes, blisters, dryness, itching, and discolored patches.

Management: Maintaining good hygiene, keeping the skin moisturized, and managing blood sugar levels are essential. Prompt treatment of infections and skin issues is also important.

# The Importance of Early Detection and Management

Early detection and effective management of diabetes are critical to preventing or delaying the onset of complications. Here are some key strategies for managing diabetes:

## Regular Monitoring:

Frequent monitoring of blood sugar levels helps in making timely adjustments to diet, medication, and lifestyle. Continuous glucose monitors (CGMs) and self-monitoring tools are valuable for tracking blood sugar trends.

## Healthy Eating:

A balanced diet rich in whole grains, fruits, vegetables, lean proteins, and healthy fats can help manage blood sugar levels. Understanding the glycemic index of foods and practicing portion control are essential.

## Physical Activity:

Regular exercise improves insulin sensitivity, aids in weight management, and enhances overall cardiovascular health. Activities such as walking, cycling, swimming, and strength training are beneficial.

## Medication Adherence:

Taking prescribed medications, including insulin and oral hypoglycemic agents, as directed by a healthcare provider is crucial for maintaining blood sugar control.

## Regular Check-ups:

Routine visits to healthcare providers for comprehensive diabetes management, including eye exams, foot exams, and screening for complications, are essential.

## Education and Support:

Diabetes education programs and support groups provide valuable information and emotional support. Learning about diabetes self-management can empower individuals to take control of their health.

## Stress Management:

Chronic stress can negatively impact blood sugar levels. Techniques such as mindfulness, meditation, yoga, and deep breathing exercises can help manage stress.

# 1.3 Conventional Treatments vs. Natural Remedies

Diabetes is a chronic condition characterized by high levels of sugar (glucose) in the blood. Managing diabetes effectively is crucial to prevent complications such as heart disease, kidney failure, and vision loss. Traditional medical approaches and natural remedies both offer pathways to manage diabetes, each with its own set of advantages and limitations. In this section, we will explore both conventional treatments and natural remedies, comparing their methodologies, benefits, and potential drawbacks.

## Conventional Treatments for Diabetes

Conventional treatments for diabetes are primarily focused on regulating blood sugar levels through medication, diet, and lifestyle changes. These treatments are evidence-based and widely accepted by the medical community.

# Medications

Insulin Therapy:

Purpose: Insulin therapy is essential for individuals with Type 1 diabetes, where the body fails to produce insulin. It is also used in some cases of Type 2 diabetes when other treatments are not sufficient.

Types of Insulin: Rapid-acting, short-acting, intermediate-acting, and long-acting insulin. Each type works at different speeds and durations to control blood sugar.

Administration: Insulin is typically administered through injections or an insulin pump. Dosages are personalized based on individual needs.

## Oral Hypoglycemic Agents:

Metformin: Often the first line of treatment for Type 2 diabetes, Metformin reduces glucose production in the liver and improves insulin sensitivity.

Sulfonylureas: These stimulate the pancreas to produce more insulin.

DPP-4 Inhibitors: These help increase insulin release and decrease glucagon levels.

SGLT2 Inhibitors: These medications help the kidneys remove excess glucose through urine.

## GLP-1 Receptor Agonists:

Purpose: These injectable medications enhance insulin secretion, suppress glucagon, slow gastric emptying, and promote satiety, leading to weight loss.

## Lifestyle Modifications

### Diet:

Carbohydrate Counting: Managing the intake of carbohydrates to prevent spikes in blood sugar.

Balanced Diet: Emphasizing whole grains, fruits, vegetables, lean proteins, and healthy fats while minimizing sugary and processed foods.

Glycemic Index: Choosing foods with a low glycemic index that have a slower impact on blood sugar levels.

Exercise:

Regular Physical Activity: Engaging in at least 150 minutes of moderate-intensity exercise per week helps improve insulin sensitivity and overall glucose control.

Strength Training: Building muscle mass can improve glucose utilization.

Weight Management:

Achieving a Healthy Weight: Weight loss can significantly improve blood sugar control and reduce the need for medications in Type 2 diabetes.

Monitoring Blood Sugar:

Self-Monitoring: Regularly checking blood glucose levels helps individuals understand how different foods, activities, and medications affect their blood sugar.

HbA1c Test: A blood test that provides average blood glucose levels over the past 2-3 months, guiding long-term treatment plans.

## Natural Remedies for Diabetes

Natural remedies for diabetes focus on holistic approaches, including dietary changes, herbal supplements, and lifestyle modifications. These methods aim to manage and potentially reverse diabetes by addressing its root causes rather than just symptoms.

Dietary Changes

Whole Foods Diet:

Plant-Based Eating: Emphasizing vegetables, fruits, nuts, seeds, legumes, and whole grains to provide essential nutrients and fiber.

Minimizing Processed Foods: Avoiding foods high in refined sugars and unhealthy fats.

Low-Carbohydrate Diet:

Ketogenic Diet: High-fat, moderate-protein, and very low-carbohydrate diet that shifts the body's metabolism to burn fat for energy instead of glucose.

Benefits: Can lead to significant improvements in blood sugar control and weight loss.

Intermittent Fasting:

Eating Patterns: Alternating periods of eating and fasting to improve insulin sensitivity and reduce blood sugar levels.

Herbal Supplements

Bitter Melon:

Properties: Contains compounds that mimic insulin and lower blood sugar levels.

Usage: Can be consumed as a juice, supplement, or in cooked dishes.

Fenugreek:

Benefits: Rich in soluble fiber, which helps lower blood sugar by slowing digestion and absorption of carbohydrates.

Forms: Seeds can be used in cooking, soaked in water, or taken as supplements.

Cinnamon:

Effects: Improves insulin sensitivity and lowers fasting blood sugar levels.

Incorporation: Can be added to meals, beverages, or taken as an extract.

Aloe Vera:

Role: May enhance insulin sensitivity and improve blood glucose management.

Consumption: Usually taken as a supplement or in aloe vera juice form.

Berberine:

Mechanism: Activates an enzyme called AMPK, which helps regulate metabolism and blood sugar levels.

Sources: Found in plants like goldenseal, barberry, and Oregon grape.

## Lifestyle Modifications

Regular Physical Activity:

Holistic Approach: Combining cardiovascular exercises, strength training, and flexibility exercises like yoga.

Benefits: Enhances insulin sensitivity and overall health.

Stress Management:

Techniques: Mindfulness meditation, deep breathing exercises, and progressive muscle relaxation.

Impact: Reduces stress hormones that can negatively affect blood sugar control.

Adequate Sleep:

Importance: Quality sleep is crucial for maintaining hormonal balance and insulin sensitivity.

Strategies: Establishing a regular sleep schedule, creating a restful environment, and avoiding stimulants before bedtime.

Hydration:

Water Intake: Staying well-hydrated helps the kidneys flush out excess glucose through urine.

Herbal Teas: Consuming herbal teas like green tea, which may have additional blood sugar-lowering effects.

Comparing Conventional Treatments and Natural Remedies

Effectiveness:

Conventional Treatments: Backed by extensive research and clinical trials, providing predictable outcomes.

Natural Remedies: Growing body of evidence supports their benefits, but individual results can vary, and more research is needed.

Safety and Side Effects:

Conventional Treatments: Medications can have side effects and require careful monitoring and adjustments by healthcare providers.

Natural Remedies: Generally considered safe when used appropriately, but interactions with medications and potential side effects should be considered.

Accessibility:

Conventional Treatments: Widely available and covered by many health insurance plans.

Natural Remedies: Accessibility may vary based on location, and some supplements can be costly.

Holistic Approach:

Conventional Treatments: Focuses on symptom management and preventing complications.

Natural Remedies: Emphasizes overall health, addressing the root causes of diabetes and promoting a holistic lifestyle.

## Integrating Conventional and Natural Approaches

Many individuals find that a combination of conventional treatments and natural remedies offers the best results. Working with healthcare providers to create a personalized plan that incorporates both approaches can help manage diabetes effectively and improve overall well-being.

### Consultation:

Healthcare Provider: Regular consultations with doctors to monitor progress and adjust treatments as needed.

Holistic Practitioners: Seeking advice from nutritionists, herbalists, or naturopaths for natural remedies.

Balanced Approach:

Medication and Herbs: Using herbal supplements alongside prescribed medications to enhance blood sugar control.

Diet and Exercise: Combining dietary changes with conventional dietary advice and incorporating regular physical activity.

Monitoring:

Self-Monitoring: Keeping track of blood sugar levels, dietary intake, and physical activity to identify patterns and adjust strategies.

Professional Monitoring: Regular health check-ups and lab tests to ensure overall health and safety.

# Chapter 2: The Role of Diet in Managing Diabetes

## 2.1 The Science of Nutrition and Diabetes

### Understanding the Connection

Diabetes, a chronic condition characterized by high blood sugar levels, is profoundly influenced by diet. To manage diabetes effectively, it is crucial to understand how nutrition impacts blood sugar regulation and overall health. The foods we consume directly affect blood glucose levels, insulin sensitivity, and weight management, all of which are critical components in diabetes management.

## How Food Affects Blood Sugar Levels

When we eat, our bodies break down carbohydrates into glucose, which enters the bloodstream. In response, the pancreas releases insulin, a hormone that allows cells to absorb glucose for energy. In individuals with diabetes, this process is disrupted. In type 1 diabetes, the body does not produce insulin, while in type 2 diabetes, the body either does not produce enough insulin or becomes resistant to its effects.

The type, amount, and timing of carbohydrate intake are key factors in managing blood sugar levels. Foods high in simple carbohydrates, like sugary snacks and refined grains, cause rapid spikes in blood glucose. Conversely, complex carbohydrates, such as whole grains and vegetables, break down more slowly, leading to gradual increases in blood sugar. Understanding these dynamics helps in planning meals that maintain stable blood glucose levels.

## The Glycemic Index and Load

The Glycemic Index (GI) is a tool that ranks foods based on their impact on blood sugar levels. Foods with a high GI cause quick spikes in blood sugar, while those with a low GI lead to slower, more sustained increases. Examples of high GI foods include white bread and sugary cereals, whereas low GI foods include legumes, most fruits, and non-starchy vegetables.

Glycemic Load (GL) takes the GI concept a step further by considering the quantity of carbohydrates in a portion of food. It provides a more accurate picture of a food's impact on blood sugar. For example, watermelon has a high GI but a low GL due to its high water content and low carbohydrate density.

Using GI and GL to guide food choices can be beneficial in managing diabetes. Incorporating more low-GI foods helps in maintaining stable blood glucose levels and preventing spikes.

## Macronutrients: Carbohydrates, Proteins, and Fats

A balanced diet for diabetes management includes appropriate proportions of carbohydrates, proteins, and fats.

Carbohydrates: Despite their impact on blood sugar, carbohydrates are a necessary part of the diet. The key is choosing the right types and amounts. Focus on whole grains, legumes, vegetables, and fruits. Aim for a consistent intake throughout the day to avoid large fluctuations in blood glucose.

Proteins: Proteins have a minimal effect on blood sugar levels and are essential for muscle repair and immune function. Good sources include lean meats, poultry, fish, eggs, dairy, legumes, nuts, and seeds. Including protein in every meal can help in maintaining satiety and stabilizing blood sugar.

Fats: Healthy fats, such as those from avocados, nuts, seeds, and olive oil, support heart health and provide long-lasting energy. Avoid trans fats and limit saturated fats, as they can increase the risk of cardiovascular disease, which is a concern for individuals with diabetes.

Micronutrients: Vitamins and Minerals

Micronutrients play a crucial role in overall health and diabetes management. Certain vitamins and minerals are particularly important:

Vitamin D: Helps in maintaining bone health and has been linked to improved insulin sensitivity. Sources include sunlight exposure, fortified foods, and supplements.

Magnesium: Involved in over 300 enzymatic reactions, including those related to glucose metabolism. Found in green leafy vegetables, nuts, seeds, and whole grains.

Chromium: Enhances insulin action and is found in whole grains, nuts, and broccoli.

Omega-3 Fatty Acids: Found in fatty fish, flaxseeds, and walnuts, these fats help reduce inflammation and improve heart health.

Ensuring a diet rich in these and other essential nutrients supports overall well-being and aids in the effective management of diabetes.

## Common Dietary Myths and Misconceptions

Several myths and misconceptions about diet and diabetes persist, leading to confusion and potentially harmful choices.

Myth 1: Diabetics Should Avoid All Carbohydrates: While it is important to manage carbohydrate intake, completely avoiding them is unnecessary and impractical. The focus should be on the quality and quantity of carbohydrates, emphasizing whole, minimally processed sources.

Myth 2: Sugar is the Only Culprit: Although sugar significantly impacts blood glucose levels, other factors, such as overall calorie intake, portion sizes, and the type of carbohydrates consumed, also play crucial roles. Complex carbohydrates and fiber-rich foods should be prioritized.

Myth 3: Diabetic Foods are Essential: Many products marketed as "diabetic-friendly" are not necessarily healthier. They may contain sugar substitutes, unhealthy fats, or excessive calories. It is better to focus on whole, nutrient-dense foods.

Myth 4: Protein and Fat Have No Impact on Blood Sugar: While protein and fat do not cause immediate blood sugar spikes, they can affect blood glucose indirectly. High-fat meals can slow down carbohydrate absorption, leading to delayed spikes, and excessive protein can be converted to glucose in the body.

# Introduction to Dr. Barbara O'Neill's Approach

Dr. Barbara O'Neill advocates a holistic approach to diabetes management, emphasizing the power of nutrition and herbal remedies. Her philosophy integrates scientific understanding with natural healing practices, offering a comprehensive strategy for managing and potentially reversing diabetes.

## Overview of Dr. Barbara's Philosophy

Dr. Barbara believes that the body has an innate ability to heal itself when provided with the right tools. Her approach focuses on:

Whole Foods: Consuming nutrient-dense, minimally processed foods that support overall health and stable blood sugar levels.

Herbal Remedies: Utilizing herbs with medicinal properties to enhance insulin sensitivity, reduce blood sugar levels, and improve overall health.

Lifestyle Changes: Incorporating regular physical activity, stress management, and sufficient sleep to support diabetes management.

## The Role of Herbal Remedies in Diabetes Management

Herbal remedies have been used for centuries to treat various ailments, including diabetes. Dr. Barbara O'Neill's approach includes specific herbs known for their beneficial effects on blood sugar levels. These herbs can complement a healthy diet and lifestyle, providing additional support for managing diabetes.

Key Herbs in Dr. Barbara's Approach

Bitter Melon: Known for its hypoglycemic properties, bitter melon can help lower blood sugar levels. It contains compounds that mimic insulin and enhance glucose uptake by cells.

Fenugreek: Rich in soluble fiber, fenugreek helps slow down the digestion and absorption of carbohydrates, leading to more stable blood sugar levels.

Cinnamon: This spice has been shown to improve insulin sensitivity and lower blood sugar levels. Including cinnamon in the diet can be a simple yet effective strategy.

Gymnema Sylvestre: Often referred to as the "sugar destroyer," this herb reduces sugar absorption in the intestines and enhances insulin function.

Other Herbs: Aloe vera, berberine, and ginseng are also part of Dr. Barbara's herbal toolkit for managing diabetes.

# Chapter 2.2 Nutritional Requirements for Diabetics

Understanding the nutritional requirements for diabetics is crucial in managing blood sugar levels and preventing complications associated with diabetes. Proper nutrition can help maintain optimal blood glucose levels, support overall health, and reduce the risk of chronic conditions. This section will explore the essential macronutrients and micronutrients needed for diabetics, providing detailed information on their roles, sources, and how to incorporate them into a diabetes-friendly diet.

## Macronutrients: Carbohydrates, Proteins, and Fats

Carbohydrates

Carbohydrates are the primary source of energy for the body, but they have the most significant impact on blood sugar levels. Therefore, managing carbohydrate intake is a critical aspect of diabetes management.

Types of Carbohydrates: There are three main types of carbohydrates – sugars, starches, and fibers. Sugars are simple carbohydrates found in fruits, vegetables, and dairy products. Starches are complex carbohydrates found in grains, legumes, and starchy vegetables. Fiber is a type of complex carbohydrate that the body cannot digest, found in fruits, vegetables, whole grains, and legumes.

Glycemic Index (GI): The glycemic index measures how quickly carbohydrates in food raise blood sugar levels. Foods with a high GI cause rapid spikes in blood sugar, while low-GI foods result in slower, steadier increases. Diabetics should focus on low to moderate GI foods, such as whole grains, legumes, non-starchy vegetables, and most fruits.

Portion Control: Managing portion sizes is essential for controlling carbohydrate intake. Diabetics should aim for consistent carbohydrate intake throughout the day, divided into small, balanced meals and snacks. A registered dietitian can help develop an individualized meal plan that aligns with personal preferences and blood sugar goals.

Proteins

Proteins are essential for building and repairing tissues, producing enzymes and hormones, and supporting immune function. While proteins have a minimal impact on blood sugar levels, they play a crucial role in overall health.

Sources of Protein: Lean meats, poultry, fish, eggs, dairy products, legumes, nuts, and seeds are excellent sources of protein. Including a variety of protein sources in the diet ensures an adequate intake of essential amino acids.

Protein and Satiety: Protein can increase feelings of fullness and reduce overall calorie intake, which can help with weight management. This is particularly beneficial for diabetics, as maintaining a healthy weight can improve insulin sensitivity and blood sugar control.

Balancing Protein Intake: While protein is essential, excessive intake can strain the kidneys, especially in individuals with diabetic nephropathy (kidney disease). It's important to consume protein in moderation and consult with a healthcare provider to determine the appropriate amount based on individual needs.

Fats

Fats are a concentrated source of energy and are vital for absorbing fat-soluble vitamins (A, D, E, and K), protecting organs, and supporting cell function. The type and amount of fat consumed can significantly impact heart health, which is a major concern for diabetics.

Types of Fats: There are four main types of fats – saturated fats, trans fats, monounsaturated fats, and polyunsaturated fats. Saturated and trans fats can raise LDL (bad) cholesterol levels, increasing the risk of heart disease. These fats are found in fatty meats, full-fat dairy products, fried foods, and many processed snacks. Monounsaturated and polyunsaturated fats can lower LDL cholesterol and are beneficial for heart health. These fats are found in olive oil, avocados, nuts, seeds, and fatty fish like salmon and mackerel.

Omega-3 Fatty Acids: Omega-3 fatty acids, a type of polyunsaturated fat, have anti-inflammatory properties and can reduce the risk of heart disease. They are found in fatty fish, flaxseeds, chia seeds, and walnuts. Including omega-3-rich foods in the diet is particularly beneficial for diabetics.

Balancing Fat Intake: Diabetics should focus on consuming healthy fats while limiting saturated and trans fats. Incorporating sources of monounsaturated and polyunsaturated fats, such as nuts, seeds, and olive oil, can help improve lipid profiles and support overall health.

## Micronutrients: Vitamins and Minerals

Micronutrients, including vitamins and minerals, are essential for various bodily functions, including metabolism, immune function, and bone health. Diabetics have specific micronutrient needs that must be met to support blood sugar control and overall health.

## Vitamins

Vitamin D: Vitamin D is crucial for bone health, immune function, and insulin sensitivity. Diabetics often have lower levels of vitamin D, which can affect blood sugar control. Sources of vitamin D include sunlight exposure, fatty fish, fortified dairy products, and supplements.

Vitamin B12: Vitamin B12 is essential for nerve function and red blood cell production. Metformin, a common medication for type 2 diabetes, can reduce B12 absorption, leading to deficiency. Sources of vitamin B12 include meat, poultry, fish, dairy products, and fortified cereals.

Antioxidant Vitamins (C and E): Vitamins C and E have antioxidant properties that can reduce oxidative stress and inflammation, which are common in diabetics. Vitamin C is found in citrus fruits, berries, and vegetables, while vitamin E is found in nuts, seeds, and vegetable oils.

Minerals

Magnesium: Magnesium plays a role in glucose metabolism and insulin sensitivity. Diabetics often have lower magnesium levels, which can affect blood sugar control. Sources of magnesium include leafy greens, nuts, seeds, whole grains, and legumes.

Chromium: Chromium is involved in carbohydrate and lipid metabolism and enhances insulin action. While deficiency is rare, adequate intake can support blood sugar control. Sources of chromium include whole grains, nuts, broccoli, and meats.

Zinc: Zinc is essential for immune function, wound healing, and insulin synthesis. Diabetics may have lower zinc levels, affecting these processes. Sources of zinc include meat, shellfish, legumes, seeds, and nuts.

# Practical Tips for Meeting Nutritional Requirements

Balanced Meals

Creating balanced meals that include a variety of macronutrients and micronutrients is crucial for managing diabetes. A balanced plate should consist of:

Half non-starchy vegetables (e.g., leafy greens, broccoli, peppers)

One-quarter lean protein (e.g., chicken, fish, tofu)

One-quarter whole grains or starchy vegetables (e.g., brown rice, quinoa, sweet potatoes)

Portion Control

Using portion control strategies can help manage calorie intake and prevent blood sugar spikes. Practical tips include:

Using smaller plates and bowls to control portions

Measuring servings with cups or a food scale

Reading nutrition labels to understand serving sizes

Regular Monitoring

Regularly monitoring blood sugar levels can help diabetics understand how different foods affect their blood sugar. Keeping a food diary and noting blood sugar readings can provide valuable insights and help make necessary dietary adjustments.

## Hydration

Staying hydrated is important for overall health and can aid in blood sugar control. Diabetics should aim to drink plenty of water throughout the day and limit sugary beverages, which can cause blood sugar spikes.

## Consulting Professionals

Working with healthcare professionals, such as registered dietitians and certified diabetes educators, can provide personalized guidance and support. These professionals can help create individualized meal plans, address specific nutritional needs, and offer strategies for managing diabetes effectively.

# 2.3 Common Dietary Myths and Misconceptions

When it comes to managing diabetes, there is a plethora of information available. Unfortunately, not all of it is accurate. Misconceptions and myths about diet and diabetes can lead to confusion, making it harder for individuals to manage their condition effectively. In this chapter, we will debunk some of the most common dietary myths and provide clear, evidence-based information to help you make informed choices.

## Myth 1: Diabetics Should Avoid All Carbohydrates

**The Truth: Not All Carbohydrates Are Created Equal**

One of the most pervasive myths is that people with diabetes should avoid all carbohydrates. While it's true that carbohydrates have a significant impact on blood sugar levels, it's not necessary (or healthy) to eliminate them entirely from your diet. Carbohydrates are an essential macronutrient that provides energy for the body.

What matters more is the type and quantity of carbohydrates you consume. Complex carbohydrates, such as those found in whole grains, vegetables, and legumes, are absorbed more slowly and have a gentler effect on blood sugar levels compared to simple carbohydrates like white bread, sugary snacks, and soda. By focusing on whole, unprocessed foods and paying attention to portion sizes, diabetics can enjoy carbohydrates as part of a balanced diet.

Key Points:

Choose complex carbohydrates over simple ones.

Monitor portion sizes to avoid spikes in blood sugar.

Include a variety of carbohydrates from whole foods.

## Myth 2: Sugar is the Sole Cause of Diabetes

**The Truth: Multiple Factors Contribute to Diabetes**

Another widespread misconception is that consuming sugar is the only cause of diabetes. While excessive sugar intake can contribute to obesity, which is a risk factor for type 2 diabetes, it is not the sole cause. Diabetes is a complex condition influenced by various factors, including genetics, lifestyle, and overall diet.

Type 1 diabetes is an autoimmune condition where the body's immune system attacks the insulin-producing cells in the pancreas. Type 2 diabetes, on the other hand, is more closely linked to lifestyle factors, such as being overweight or obese, physical inactivity, and poor diet. While it's important for diabetics to monitor their sugar intake, focusing solely on sugar overlooks the broader picture of a healthy diet and lifestyle.

Key Points:

Diabetes is influenced by a combination of factors, not just sugar consumption.

Maintaining a balanced diet and healthy lifestyle is crucial for managing diabetes.

Focus on overall dietary patterns rather than isolating sugar as the sole culprit.

## Myth 3: Fruit is Off-Limits for Diabetics

### The Truth: Fruit Can Be Part of a Healthy Diabetic Diet

Many people with diabetes believe they must avoid fruit because of its natural sugar content. However, fruits are packed with essential vitamins, minerals, and fiber, making them a valuable part of a healthy diet. The key is to choose fruits with a lower glycemic index (GI) and monitor portion sizes to keep blood sugar levels stable.

Fruits such as berries, apples, and pears have a lower GI and are less likely to cause spikes in blood sugar. Pairing fruit with a source of protein or healthy fat, such as nuts or yogurt, can also help mitigate its impact on blood sugar levels. It's important for diabetics to enjoy fruit in moderation and be mindful of how it fits into their overall carbohydrate intake for the day.

Key Points:

Fruits provide essential nutrients and fiber.

Choose low-GI fruits and monitor portion sizes.

Pair fruit with protein or fat to stabilize blood sugar levels.

## Myth 4: Diabetics Must Eat Special "Diabetic" Foods

### The Truth: Healthy Eating is Universal

The market is flooded with products labeled as "diabetic-friendly" or "sugar-free," leading many to believe that they must consume these special foods to manage their diabetes. However, many of these products are highly processed and can contain unhealthy ingredients, such as artificial sweeteners and trans fats.

A healthy diet for diabetics is fundamentally the same as a healthy diet for anyone else: it should be rich in whole foods, such as vegetables, fruits, whole grains, lean proteins, and healthy fats. Instead of relying on specially labeled products, focus on natural, minimally processed foods. Reading nutrition labels and being aware of ingredients can help you make healthier choices without falling into the trap of "diabetic" marketing.

Key Points:

Avoid highly processed "diabetic" foods.

Focus on a balanced diet rich in whole, minimally processed foods.

Read nutrition labels to make informed choices.

## Myth 5: You Can't Enjoy Your Favorite Foods

### The Truth: Moderation and Balance Are Key

Managing diabetes does not mean you have to give up all your favorite foods. The key is moderation and balance. It's possible to enjoy occasional treats or indulgent meals by making smart choices and planning ahead.

For instance, if you know you will be having a higher-carb meal or a dessert, you can adjust your other meals and snacks throughout the day to balance your carbohydrate intake. Using portion control and finding healthier ways to prepare your favorite dishes can also help you enjoy them without negatively impacting your blood sugar levels. Remember, the goal is to create a sustainable, enjoyable way of eating that supports your health and well-being.

Key Points:

Enjoy favorite foods in moderation.

Balance higher-carb meals with lower-carb options.

Use portion control and healthier preparation methods.

## Myth 6: All Fats Are Bad for Diabetics

### The Truth: Healthy Fats Are Beneficial

Fats have often been vilified in discussions about healthy eating, but not all fats are bad. In fact, healthy fats, such as those found in avocados, nuts, seeds, and olive oil, can be beneficial for diabetics. These fats can help improve heart health, which is particularly important for people with diabetes, who are at higher risk for cardiovascular disease.

Trans fats and saturated fats, found in processed foods and fatty cuts of meat, should be limited, as they can raise cholesterol levels and increase the risk of heart disease. Including healthy fats in your diet can help you feel satisfied and support overall health without negatively impacting blood sugar levels.

Key Points:

Include healthy fats from sources like avocados, nuts, seeds, and olive oil.

Limit trans fats and saturated fats.

Healthy fats can support heart health and overall well-being.

## Myth 7: Protein Has No Impact on Blood Sugar

The Truth: Protein Affects Blood Sugar Indirectly

While protein doesn't raise blood sugar levels as quickly or significantly as carbohydrates, it still plays a role in blood sugar management. High-protein diets can influence insulin sensitivity and satiety, which can indirectly affect blood sugar control.

Including adequate protein in your diet can help stabilize blood sugar levels by slowing the absorption of carbohydrates. It can also help maintain muscle mass, which is important for overall health and metabolism. Balance is key, and it's important to choose lean protein sources, such as fish, poultry, beans, and legumes, while avoiding high-fat and processed protein sources.

Key Points:

Protein affects blood sugar indirectly.

Include adequate protein to stabilize blood sugar and support muscle health.

Choose lean protein sources and avoid processed options.

# Chapter 2.4: Introduction to Dr. Barbara O'Neill's Approach

Dr. Barbara O'Neill is a renowned naturopath, nutritionist, and author, widely recognized for her expertise in natural health and wellness. Her approach to managing diabetes centers on holistic principles, emphasizing the importance of diet, lifestyle changes, and the use of herbal remedies. In this section, we will delve into Dr. Barbara's philosophy, the role of herbal remedies in diabetes management, and how her approach can be integrated into a practical and sustainable lifestyle.

Dr. Barbara O'Neill's Philosophy

Dr. Barbara O'Neill's philosophy is rooted in the belief that the body has an inherent ability to heal itself when given the right conditions. This belief is the cornerstone of her approach to managing and potentially reversing diabetes. She advocates for a natural, holistic lifestyle that prioritizes whole foods, physical activity, stress management, and the use of natural remedies.

One of the key tenets of Dr. Barbara's philosophy is the idea that many chronic diseases, including diabetes, are largely influenced by lifestyle choices. She emphasizes the need to address the root causes of the disease rather than merely treating its symptoms. This involves making significant changes to diet, incorporating regular physical activity, managing stress, and utilizing the healing properties of herbs and other natural substances.

Dr. Barbara also places a strong emphasis on education and empowerment. She believes that individuals should be well-informed about their health and the impact of their choices. By providing comprehensive education on nutrition, natural remedies, and lifestyle changes, she empowers individuals to take control of their health and make informed decisions.

## The Role of Herbal Remedies in Diabetes Management

Herbal remedies have been used for centuries in various cultures to treat a wide range of ailments, including diabetes. Dr. Barbara O'Neill incorporates these time-honored practices into her approach, using specific herbs known for their beneficial effects on blood sugar levels and overall health. Here, we will explore some of the key herbs she recommends and how they can be integrated into a diabetes management plan.

Bitter Melon (Momordica charantia)

Properties: Bitter melon is rich in compounds that have been shown to lower blood sugar levels. It contains charantin, vicine, and polypeptide-p, which mimic insulin's effects.

Usage: Bitter melon can be consumed in various forms, including fresh juice, cooked dishes, and supplements. It is often recommended to start with small amounts and gradually increase the dosage to avoid gastrointestinal discomfort.

Fenugreek (Trigonella foenum-graecum)

Properties: Fenugreek seeds are high in soluble fiber, which helps regulate blood sugar levels by slowing down the absorption of carbohydrates. They also contain compounds that stimulate insulin secretion.

Usage: Fenugreek seeds can be soaked in water overnight and consumed on an empty stomach, ground into powder and added to meals, or taken as supplements.

Cinnamon (Cinnamomum verum)

Properties: Cinnamon has been shown to improve insulin sensitivity and lower blood sugar levels. It contains cinnamaldehyde, which has anti-inflammatory and antioxidant properties.

Usage: Cinnamon can be added to a variety of dishes, including oatmeal, smoothies, and baked goods. It is important to use Ceylon cinnamon, also known as "true" cinnamon, as it has lower levels of coumarin, a compound that can be harmful                    in                    large                    amounts.

Gymnema Sylvestre

Properties: Gymnema sylvestre has been traditionally used in Ayurvedic medicine for its anti-diabetic properties. It helps reduce sugar absorption in the intestines and enhances insulin production.

Usage: Gymnema sylvestre can be taken in the form of capsules, powders, or teas. It is often recommended to consult a healthcare provider before starting Gymnema sylvestre, especially for those on diabetes medication.

Other Effective Herbs

Aloe Vera: Known for its soothing properties, aloe vera also helps lower blood glucose levels. It can be consumed as juice or supplements.

Ginseng: Both American and Asian ginseng have been shown to improve insulin sensitivity and reduce blood sugar levels. Ginseng is available in various forms, including teas, capsules, and extracts.

Berberine: Found in several plants, berberine has powerful blood sugar-lowering effects. It is typically taken in supplement form.

Integrating Herbal Remedies into Your Diet

Incorporating herbal remedies into your daily routine can be straightforward and enjoyable. Here are some practical tips on how to do so:

## Herbal Teas and Infusions

Herbal teas are an easy way to include beneficial herbs in your diet. For instance, you can brew a tea using dried fenugreek seeds or Gymnema sylvestre leaves. Drinking these teas regularly can help manage blood sugar levels.

## Herbal Supplements and Extracts

If you prefer not to prepare herbal teas, supplements and extracts are convenient alternatives. These are widely available in health food stores and online. Always choose high-quality products and follow the recommended dosages.

### Cooking with Herbs

Many of these herbs can be integrated into your cooking. For example, add cinnamon to your morning oatmeal, use fenugreek seeds in your curries, or incorporate bitter melon into stir-fries. This not only enhances the flavor of your meals but also provides health benefits.

### Combining Herbs

Some herbs work synergistically when combined. For instance, a mixture of cinnamon and Gymnema sylvestre can provide a potent blood sugar-lowering effect. Experiment with different combinations to find what works best for you.

### Safety and Efficacy of Herbal Remedies

While herbal remedies can be highly effective in managing diabetes, it is crucial to use them safely. Here are some guidelines to ensure their safe and effective use:

Consult with Healthcare Providers

Before starting any new herbal remedy, consult with your healthcare provider, especially if you are taking medications or have other health conditions. Some herbs can interact with medications, leading to adverse effects.

Start with Small Doses

Begin with small doses and gradually increase as needed. This helps your body adjust to the new herb and reduces the risk of side effects.

Monitor Blood Sugar Levels

Regularly monitor your blood sugar levels to assess the effectiveness of the herbal remedies. Keep a log of your readings and any changes in your symptoms.

Be Aware of Potential Side Effects

Some herbs can cause side effects, such as gastrointestinal discomfort or allergic reactions. If you experience any adverse effects, discontinue use and consult your healthcare provider.

Choose High-Quality Products

Ensure you are using high-quality herbs and supplements. Look for products that are certified organic, non-GMO, and free from contaminants.

# Chapter 3: Dr. Barbara O'Neill's Herbal Remedies

## 3.1 The Healing Power of Herbs

Herbal remedies have been used for thousands of years across various cultures to treat a multitude of ailments. In the context of diabetes, these natural treatments offer a complementary approach to conventional medicine, potentially aiding in the management and reduction of symptoms. Dr. Barbara O'Neill, a prominent figure in the field of natural health, advocates for the use of specific herbs in diabetes management. Understanding the healing power of these herbs can empower individuals to take control of their health in a natural and effective way.

## Historical Use of Herbs in Medicine

Herbal medicine has a rich history that dates back to ancient civilizations. The Egyptians, Chinese, Greeks, and Native Americans, among others, have utilized plants for their medicinal properties. For instance, the ancient Egyptians documented the use of herbs such as garlic and coriander in their medical papyri. Traditional Chinese Medicine (TCM) has a comprehensive system that incorporates herbs like ginseng and astragalus to balance the body's energy and treat illnesses.

In the context of diabetes, traditional Indian Ayurveda has long recognized the benefits of certain herbs in managing blood sugar levels. Herbs such as fenugreek and bitter melon have been staples in Ayurvedic practices, reflecting a deep understanding of their therapeutic properties.

## Modern Research on Herbal Remedies

Modern scientific research has validated many of the traditional uses of herbs, demonstrating their potential in managing various health conditions, including diabetes. Research has shown that certain herbs can help regulate blood sugar levels, enhance insulin sensitivity, and reduce inflammation—key factors in the management of diabetes.

Studies have indicated that bitter melon, for instance, contains compounds that mimic insulin, which can help lower blood sugar levels. Similarly, cinnamon has been shown to improve insulin sensitivity and reduce fasting blood sugar levels in individuals with type 2 diabetes. The convergence of traditional wisdom and modern science underscores the efficacy of these herbal remedies.

## Essential Herbs for Diabetes Management

Dr. Barbara O'Neill highlights several key herbs that are particularly effective in managing diabetes. These herbs have been extensively studied and are known for their blood sugar-lowering properties.

Bitter Melon (Momordica charantia)

Bitter melon, also known as bitter gourd, is a tropical vine widely used in Asia and Africa. It contains active substances such as charantin, vicine, and polypeptide-p, which have been shown to have hypoglycemic effects. Bitter melon works by increasing the uptake of glucose by cells, enhancing insulin secretion, and inhibiting enzymes that break down carbohydrates into glucose.

Usage: Bitter melon can be consumed as a juice, tea, or incorporated into various dishes. It is important to start with small amounts and gradually increase the dosage to avoid gastrointestinal discomfort.

Fenugreek (Trigonella foenum-graecum)

Fenugreek seeds are a common spice in Indian cuisine, known for their distinct flavor and medicinal properties. They are rich in soluble fiber, which helps slow down the absorption of carbohydrates and sugars. Fenugreek seeds also contain trigonelline, a compound that has been shown to improve insulin sensitivity.

Usage: Fenugreek seeds can be soaked in water overnight and consumed on an empty stomach, ground into a powder and added to meals, or taken as a supplement.

## Cinnamon (Cinnamomum verum)

Cinnamon is a popular spice that has been used for its medicinal properties for centuries. Research has shown that cinnamon can lower fasting blood glucose levels and improve lipid profiles in individuals with diabetes. It works by enhancing insulin receptor activity and increasing glucose uptake by cells.

Usage: Cinnamon can be added to a variety of foods and beverages, such as oatmeal, smoothies, and tea. It is recommended to use Ceylon cinnamon, also known as "true" cinnamon, as it contains lower levels of coumarin, a compound that can be harmful in large amounts.

## Gymnema Sylvestre

Gymnema sylvestre is a woody climbing shrub native to India and Africa. Known as the "sugar destroyer" in Ayurvedic medicine, it contains gymnemic acids, which help reduce the absorption of sugar in the intestines and enhance insulin production.

Usage: Gymnema sylvestre can be taken in the form of capsules, tablets, or tea. It is advisable to follow the dosage instructions provided by a healthcare professional.

Other Effective Herbs

Berberine: Found in plants like goldenseal and barberry, berberine has been shown to improve insulin sensitivity and reduce glucose production in the liver.

Aloe Vera: Aloe vera juice can help lower fasting blood glucose levels and HbA1c, a marker of long-term blood sugar control.

Holy Basil (Tulsi): This adaptogenic herb helps reduce stress and inflammation, which can indirectly improve blood sugar control.

How to Incorporate Herbs into Your Diet

Incorporating these herbs into your daily routine can be simple and enjoyable. Here are some practical ways to do so:

Herbal Teas and Infusions

Herbal teas are a convenient and soothing way to consume medicinal herbs. For example, you can make a tea using dried bitter melon slices or fenugreek seeds. Simply steep the herbs in hot water for 10-15 minutes, strain, and enjoy. Adding a bit of lemon or honey can enhance the flavor.

## Herbal Supplements and Extracts

For those who prefer a more concentrated form, herbal supplements and extracts are available. These can be found in health food stores and pharmacies. It is important to choose high-quality products and follow the recommended dosages. Consulting with a healthcare provider before starting any new supplement is also advisable.

Cooking with Herbs

Integrating herbs into your meals can be both delicious and beneficial. For example, you can add ground cinnamon to your morning oatmeal or smoothie, use fenugreek seeds in curries and stews, or include bitter melon in stir-fries and soups. Experimenting with different recipes can make the process enjoyable and sustainable.

## Safety and Efficacy of Herbal Remedies

While herbs can offer significant health benefits, it is important to use them responsibly. Here are some guidelines to ensure their safe and effective use:

Potential Side Effects and Interactions

Some herbs can cause side effects or interact with medications. For example, bitter melon can cause gastrointestinal upset in some individuals, and cinnamon may interact with blood-thinning medications. It is crucial to start with small doses and monitor your body's response. If you experience any adverse effects, discontinue use and consult a healthcare professional.

Guidelines for Safe Use

Consultation: Always consult with a healthcare provider before starting any new herbal remedy, especially if you have pre-existing health conditions or are taking medications.

Quality: Choose high-quality herbs from reputable sources to ensure purity and potency.

Dosage: Follow recommended dosages and avoid excessive consumption.

Monitoring: Regularly monitor your blood sugar levels to assess the effectiveness of the herbs and make any necessary adjustments.

# 3.2 Essential Herbs for Diabetes Management

Herbal remedies have long been utilized in traditional medicine for their potential health benefits, including the management of diabetes. Dr. Barbara O'Neill, a renowned naturopath, emphasizes the importance of incorporating certain herbs into the diet to help regulate blood sugar levels and improve overall health. In this section, we will explore some of the most effective herbs for diabetes management, backed by both historical use and modern scientific research.

Bitter Melon (Momordica charantia)

Overview and Historical Use:

Bitter melon, also known as bitter gourd or karela, is a tropical fruit widely used in Asian and African traditional medicine. It is recognized for its distinctive bitter taste and is commonly consumed as a vegetable. Historically, bitter melon has been used to treat various ailments, including infections, skin conditions, and gastrointestinal issues.

Scientific Evidence:

Modern studies have shown that bitter melon contains bioactive compounds such as charantin, vicine, and polypeptide-p, which have antidiabetic properties. These compounds are believed to mimic insulin, enhance glucose uptake by cells, and reduce blood sugar levels. Research indicates that bitter melon can improve glycemic control in people with type 2 diabetes, making it a valuable addition to a diabetes-friendly diet.

How to Use:

Juice: Fresh bitter melon juice can be consumed daily. It is typically made by blending the melon and straining the juice.

Cooked: Bitter melon can be sautéed, stir-fried, or added to soups and stews.

Supplements: Bitter melon extracts and capsules are available as dietary supplements.

Fenugreek (Trigonella foenum-graecum)

Overview and Historical Use:

Fenugreek is an herb commonly used in Middle Eastern, Indian, and North African cuisines. Its seeds and leaves are both utilized in cooking and traditional medicine. Fenugreek has been historically employed to enhance lactation, improve digestion, and manage diabetes.

Scientific Evidence:

Fenugreek seeds are rich in soluble fiber, which helps slow down the absorption of carbohydrates and sugars in the digestive tract, leading to better blood sugar control. Studies have shown that fenugreek can lower blood sugar levels, improve glucose tolerance, and reduce fasting blood glucose levels. Additionally, fenugreek is known to have hypolipidemic effects, which can help manage cholesterol levels.

How to Use:

Seeds: Fenugreek seeds can be soaked in water overnight and consumed on an empty stomach. They can also be ground and added to food as a spice.

Leaves: Fresh fenugreek leaves can be used in salads, curries, and other dishes.

Supplements: Fenugreek supplements are available in various forms, including capsules, powders, and extracts.

Cinnamon (Cinnamomum verum)

Overview and Historical Use:

Cinnamon is a popular spice derived from the inner bark of trees belonging to the Cinnamomum genus. It has been used for centuries in both culinary and medicinal contexts. Traditionally, cinnamon has been employed to treat respiratory and digestive issues, as well as to improve circulation.

Scientific Evidence:

Cinnamon contains compounds such as cinnamaldehyde, which have been shown to possess insulin-like activity. Research suggests that cinnamon can improve insulin sensitivity, reduce blood sugar levels, and lower hemoglobin A1c (HbA1c) in individuals with type 2 diabetes. Additionally, cinnamon has antioxidant and anti-inflammatory properties that may benefit overall health.

How to Use:

Powder: Ground cinnamon can be added to a variety of dishes, including oatmeal, yogurt, smoothies, and baked goods.

Sticks: Cinnamon sticks can be used to infuse flavor into teas, stews, and other beverages.

Supplements: Cinnamon supplements are available in capsule and extract forms.

Gymnema Sylvestre

Overview and Historical Use:

Gymnema sylvestre is a climbing plant native to India and Africa. It has been used in Ayurvedic medicine for centuries to treat diabetes, malaria, and snakebites.

Gymnema is often referred to as "gurmar," which means "sugar destroyer" in Hindi.

Scientific Evidence:

Gymnema sylvestre contains gymnemic acids, which have been shown to suppress the taste of sweetness, reduce sugar absorption in the intestines, and enhance insulin secretion. Studies have demonstrated that Gymnema can lower blood sugar levels and improve glucose metabolism, making it a valuable herb for managing diabetes.

How to Use:

Tea: Gymnema leaves can be dried and used to make a herbal tea.

Powder: Gymnema powder can be mixed into water or smoothies.

Supplements: Gymnema supplements are available in capsule and extract forms.

Other Effective Herbs

1. Aloe Vera:

Aloe vera has been traditionally used for its healing properties. Recent studies suggest that aloe vera can help lower blood sugar levels and improve insulin sensitivity. Aloe vera juice or gel can be consumed as part of a daily regimen.

2. Berberine:

Berberine is a compound found in several plants, including goldenseal and barberry. It has been shown to improve insulin sensitivity, reduce glucose production in the liver, and lower blood sugar levels. Berberine supplements are widely available and can be incorporated into a diabetes management plan.

## 3. Holy Basil (Tulsi):

Holy basil, also known as tulsi, is a revered herb in Ayurvedic medicine. It is believed to have adaptogenic properties, helping the body manage stress and improve overall health. Studies indicate that holy basil can lower blood sugar levels and improve insulin secretion. Holy basil can be consumed as a tea or taken in supplement form.

## 4. Ginseng:

Ginseng, particularly American ginseng, has been studied for its antidiabetic properties. It is believed to improve insulin sensitivity and enhance glucose uptake by cells. Ginseng can be consumed as a tea, extract, or supplement.

## 5. Milk Thistle:

Milk thistle is known for its liver-protective properties. It contains silymarin, a compound that may help improve insulin resistance and reduce inflammation. Milk thistle supplements are available in various forms.

# Incorporating Herbs into Your Diet

Incorporating these herbs into your daily diet can be an effective way to manage diabetes naturally. Here are some practical tips:

Start Slowly: Introduce one herb at a time to monitor its effects on your body.

Consult a Professional: Always consult with a healthcare provider or a qualified herbalist before starting any new herbal regimen, especially if you are on medication or have underlying health conditions.

Diversify: Use a variety of herbs to take advantage of their different mechanisms of action.

Be Consistent: Regular use of these herbs, combined with a balanced diet and healthy lifestyle, can help achieve better blood sugar control.

Safety and Efficacy of Herbal Remedies

While many herbs offer promising benefits for diabetes management, it is crucial to use them safely:

Potential Side Effects: Some herbs can cause side effects or interact with medications. For instance, high doses of cinnamon can lead to liver damage, and Gymnema may affect the sense of taste.

Quality Matters: Choose high-quality, reputable brands to ensure the purity and potency of herbal products.

Dosage: Follow recommended dosages and avoid excessive use.

# 3.3 How to Incorporate Herbs into Your Diet

Incorporating herbs into your diet can be a simple and effective way to manage diabetes. Herbs offer a range of health benefits, including blood sugar regulation, improved digestion, and enhanced immunity. Dr. Barbara O'Neill's approach emphasizes the use of these natural remedies as part of a holistic strategy to support diabetes management. Here, we will explore various methods to integrate herbs into your daily meals and routines.

## Herbal Teas and Infusions

Herbal teas and infusions are among the easiest ways to incorporate herbs into your diet. They can be consumed throughout the day, offering both hydration and therapeutic benefits. Here are some commonly used herbs and their specific benefits for diabetes management:

## Bitter Melon Tea:

Benefits: Bitter melon has been shown to have hypoglycemic effects, meaning it can lower blood sugar levels. It contains compounds that mimic insulin and help improve glucose uptake.

Preparation: Slice fresh bitter melon and steep it in hot water for 10-15 minutes. You can also use dried bitter melon slices or powder.

## Fenugreek Tea:

Benefits: Fenugreek seeds are rich in soluble fiber, which helps control blood sugar levels by slowing down the absorption of carbohydrates. Fenugreek also enhances insulin sensitivity.

Preparation: Crush a teaspoon of fenugreek seeds and steep in hot water for 5-10 minutes. Strain and drink.

## Cinnamon Tea:

Benefits: Cinnamon has been shown to improve insulin sensitivity and lower blood sugar levels. It contains bioactive compounds that help in managing diabetes.

Preparation: Add a stick of cinnamon to boiling water and let it simmer for 10 minutes. Remove the stick and enjoy the tea.

## Gymnema Sylvestre Tea:

Benefits: Gymnema Sylvestre is known as the "sugar destroyer" because it helps reduce sugar absorption in the intestines and enhances insulin function.

Preparation: Use dried Gymnema leaves and steep in hot water for 5-10 minutes. Strain before drinking.

## Ginger Tea:

Benefits: Ginger helps improve insulin sensitivity and has anti-inflammatory properties that benefit overall health.

Preparation: Slice fresh ginger and steep in hot water for 10-15 minutes. Add lemon or honey for taste if desired.

## Herbal Supplements and Extracts

For those who may not enjoy the taste of herbal teas or have busy schedules, herbal supplements and extracts offer a convenient alternative. These concentrated forms provide the benefits of herbs without the need for preparation. Here are some popular herbal supplements and extracts:

Bitter Melon Capsules:

Usage: Take according to the manufacturer's instructions, typically one or two capsules daily. Consult with a healthcare provider before starting any new supplement.

Fenugreek Powder or Capsules:

Usage: Fenugreek powder can be added to smoothies, yogurt, or sprinkled over meals. Capsules are taken as directed, usually one or two per day.

Cinnamon Extract:

Usage: Cinnamon extract can be added to drinks, smoothies, or taken directly. It is important to use extracts that specify a high concentration of active compounds like cinnamaldehyde.

## Gymnema Sylvestre Supplements:

Usage: Available in capsule or tablet form, gymnema supplements are taken as directed, typically one or two times a day.

Ginger Capsules:

Usage: Ginger capsules can be taken daily to help manage blood sugar levels and inflammation.

Cooking with Herbs

Incorporating herbs directly into your cooking not only enhances flavor but also provides the medicinal benefits of these plants. Here are some practical ways to use herbs in everyday meals:

Bitter Melon in Stir-fries and Curries:

Recipe Idea: Sauté sliced bitter melon with garlic, onions, and a selection of vegetables. Add to curries or stir-fries for a nutrient-dense meal.

Fenugreek in Breads and Salads:

Recipe Idea: Add fenugreek leaves or seeds to whole-grain breads or sprinkle over salads. Fenugreek can also be incorporated into Indian dishes like dal and curry.

Cinnamon in Baking and Oatmeal:

Recipe Idea: Use cinnamon powder in baking recipes such as muffins, cookies, and breads. Sprinkle cinnamon over oatmeal, yogurt, or fruit salads for added flavor and health benefits.

Gymnema in Smoothies and Soups:

Recipe Idea: Add gymnema powder to smoothies or mix into soups and broths. It has a mild taste that blends well with other ingredients.

Ginger in Marinades and Stir-fries:

Recipe Idea: Use fresh ginger in marinades for meats and tofu. Grated ginger can be added to stir-fries, soups, and sauces to enhance flavor and provide health benefits.

Herbal Blends and DIY Remedies

Creating your own herbal blends and remedies can be a fun and rewarding way to manage diabetes. Here are some ideas for DIY herbal blends:

Diabetes Management Tea Blend:

Ingredients: Bitter melon, fenugreek seeds, cinnamon sticks, and ginger slices.

Preparation: Mix equal parts of each herb and store in an airtight container. Use one tablespoon of the blend per cup of hot water. Steep for 10-15 minutes, strain, and drink.

Herbal Spice Mix for Cooking:

Ingredients: Ground fenugreek, cinnamon, and ginger.

Preparation: Combine equal parts of each ground herb and store in a spice jar. Use this mix to season vegetables, meats, and grains.

Infused Herbal Oil:

Ingredients: Fresh or dried herbs such as rosemary, thyme, and garlic.

Preparation: Place herbs in a clean, dry jar and cover with olive oil. Let it sit for a week in a cool, dark place. Strain and use the infused oil for cooking or as a salad dressing.

Safety and Efficacy of Herbal Remedies

While herbs can offer significant benefits in managing diabetes, it is important to use them safely and effectively. Here are some guidelines to follow:

Consult with a Healthcare Provider:

Before starting any new herbal remedy, it is crucial to consult with a healthcare provider, especially if you are taking other medications. Some herbs can interact with medications and affect their efficacy.

Start with Small Amounts:

When introducing a new herb into your diet, start with small amounts to see how your body reacts. Gradually increase the quantity as needed.

Monitor Blood Sugar Levels:

Regularly monitor your blood sugar levels to understand how different herbs affect you. This will help you adjust your diet and herbal intake accordingly.

Use Quality Products:

Ensure that you are using high-quality herbs and supplements. Look for products that are organic, non-GMO, and have been tested for purity and potency.

Be Aware of Potential Side Effects:

Some herbs can cause side effects or allergic reactions. If you experience any adverse effects, discontinue use and consult a healthcare provider.

# Chapter 3.4: Safety and Efficacy of Herbal Remedies

Herbal remedies have been used for centuries in traditional medicine systems across the world to treat a variety of ailments, including diabetes. With the rising interest in natural and holistic approaches to health, many people with diabetes are turning to herbs as part of their management plan. While these natural remedies offer promising benefits, it is crucial to understand their safety and efficacy to ensure they are used correctly and effectively.

Understanding the Efficacy of Herbal Remedies

Efficacy refers to the ability of an herb to produce the desired therapeutic effect. For diabetes management, this means an herb's ability to help regulate blood sugar levels, improve insulin sensitivity, and support overall health. The efficacy of herbal remedies can be influenced by several factors:

Active Compounds: Different herbs contain various active compounds that contribute to their medicinal properties. For example, cinnamon contains cinnamaldehyde, which has been shown to improve insulin sensitivity. The concentration and availability of these compounds can affect the herb's efficacy.

Dosage and Formulation: The form in which an herb is consumed (e.g., tea, extract, capsule) and the dosage taken can significantly impact its effectiveness. Higher concentrations of active compounds in extracts may provide more potent effects than whole herb preparations.

Consistency and Duration of Use: Consistent and long-term use of herbal remedies is often necessary to achieve significant benefits. Unlike pharmaceutical drugs, which may produce rapid effects, herbs typically work more gradually.

Individual Variability: Responses to herbal remedies can vary widely among individuals due to genetic differences, the presence of other health conditions, and variations in diet and lifestyle.

## Evaluating the Safety of Herbal Remedies

Safety is a critical aspect of using herbal remedies, particularly for individuals with chronic conditions like diabetes. While many herbs are considered safe when used appropriately, there are several factors to consider to avoid adverse effects:

Potential Side Effects: Some herbs can cause side effects, especially when taken in large amounts or for extended periods. For example, fenugreek can cause gastrointestinal issues like diarrhea and bloating. It is essential to be aware of these potential side effects and monitor for any adverse reactions.

Herb-Drug Interactions: Herbs can interact with prescription medications, potentially altering their effects. For instance, garlic and ginseng can enhance the effects of blood-thinning medications, increasing the risk of bleeding. It is crucial to consult with a healthcare provider before combining herbal remedies with prescription drugs.

Quality and Purity: The quality of herbal products can vary significantly. Contaminants such as heavy metals, pesticides, and adulterants can pose health risks. Purchasing herbs from reputable sources that adhere to good manufacturing practices is vital to ensure their safety.

Allergic Reactions: Some individuals may be allergic to certain herbs. Symptoms of an allergic reaction can include skin rashes, itching, swelling, and difficulty breathing. If an allergic reaction occurs, discontinue use immediately and seek medical attention.

## Guidelines for Safe Use of Herbal Remedies

To safely incorporate herbal remedies into your diabetes management plan, consider the following guidelines:

Consult with Healthcare Providers: Before starting any herbal remedy, consult with your healthcare provider, especially if you are taking prescription medications or have other health conditions. They can help identify potential interactions and ensure that the herbs you choose are appropriate for your situation.

Start with Low Doses: When trying a new herb, start with a low dose to assess your body's response. Gradually increase the dose if no adverse effects occur. This approach helps minimize the risk of side effects and allows you to determine the appropriate dose for your needs.

Monitor Blood Sugar Levels: Regularly monitor your blood sugar levels when using herbal remedies to ensure they are having the desired effect. This monitoring will help you and your healthcare provider make any necessary adjustments to your treatment plan.

Use Reputable Products: Purchase herbal products from reputable sources that provide information about the quality, purity, and concentration of active ingredients. Look for products that have been independently tested for contaminants and adhere to good manufacturing practices.

Educate Yourself: Learn about the herbs you are using, including their potential benefits, side effects, and interactions. Reliable sources of information include peer-reviewed scientific studies, reputable health websites, and books by experts in herbal medicine.

# Popular Herbs for Diabetes Management and Their Safety Profiles

Bitter Melon (Momordica charantia): Bitter melon is known for its blood sugar-lowering properties. It contains compounds that mimic insulin and improve glucose uptake by cells. While generally safe, it can cause gastrointestinal issues in some individuals. Pregnant women should avoid it due to potential uterine contractions.

Fenugreek (Trigonella foenum-graecum): Fenugreek seeds are rich in soluble fiber, which helps manage blood sugar levels. They may also enhance insulin sensitivity. Common side effects include gastrointestinal discomfort. Fenugreek can interact with anticoagulants and antiplatelet drugs.

Cinnamon (Cinnamomum verum): Cinnamon has been shown to improve insulin sensitivity and lower blood sugar levels. Cassia cinnamon, the common variety, contains coumarin, which can be harmful in large amounts. Ceylon cinnamon is a safer alternative with lower coumarin levels.

Gymnema Sylvestre: This herb is often referred to as the "sugar destroyer" due to its ability to reduce sugar absorption in the intestines and enhance insulin function. It is generally considered safe, but large doses may cause hypoglycemia (low blood sugar).

Aloe Vera: Aloe vera gel may help lower blood sugar levels and improve insulin sensitivity. However, consuming large amounts of aloe latex (the yellow part of the leaf) can cause severe gastrointestinal issues and electrolyte imbalances.

# Chapter 4: Crafting a Diabetes-Friendly Meal Plan

## 4.1: Principles of Meal Planning for Diabetes

Creating a diabetes-friendly meal plan is crucial for managing blood sugar levels and overall health. A well-constructed meal plan helps maintain a stable glucose level, reduces the risk of complications, and supports weight management. This subchapter will delve into the principles of meal planning for diabetes, focusing on balancing macronutrients, portion control, and timing of meals.

## 1. Understanding Macronutrients

Macronutrients, which include carbohydrates, proteins, and fats, are the primary nutrients needed by the body in large amounts. Each macronutrient plays a distinct role in maintaining health and managing diabetes.

### a. Carbohydrates

Carbohydrates have the most significant impact on blood sugar levels. When consumed, carbohydrates break down into glucose, which enters the bloodstream and raises blood sugar levels. Therefore, managing carbohydrate intake is vital for diabetics. There are two types of carbohydrates:

Simple Carbohydrates: These are sugars found in fruits, vegetables, milk, and sweets. They are quickly digested and can cause rapid spikes in blood sugar levels.

Complex Carbohydrates: These are found in whole grains, legumes, and starchy vegetables. They are digested more slowly, leading to a gradual increase in blood sugar levels.

### b. Proteins

Proteins are essential for repairing tissues, building muscles, and maintaining a healthy immune system. They have a minimal impact on blood sugar levels and can help stabilize blood sugar when consumed with carbohydrates. Good sources of protein include lean meats, fish, poultry, eggs, dairy products, legumes, and nuts.

## c. Fats

Fats are necessary for overall health, providing energy, supporting cell growth, and protecting organs. However, not all fats are created equal. Healthy fats, such as those found in olive oil, avocados, nuts, and seeds, can help improve heart health, which is crucial for diabetics. Saturated and trans fats, found in processed foods and fatty meats, should be limited as they can increase the risk of heart disease.

## 2. Balancing Macronutrients

Balancing macronutrients involves ensuring that each meal contains the right proportions of carbohydrates, proteins, and fats. This balance helps maintain stable blood sugar levels and provides the nutrients needed for overall health.

## a. Carbohydrate Counting

Carbohydrate counting is a common method used by diabetics to manage their blood sugar levels. It involves tracking the number of carbohydrates consumed at each meal. The American Diabetes Association suggests that most diabetics aim for about 45-60 grams of carbohydrates per meal, but individual needs may vary.

## b. The Plate Method

The plate method is a simple way to visualize a balanced meal. It involves dividing a plate into three sections:

Half of the Plate: Non-starchy vegetables (e.g., leafy greens, broccoli, peppers)

One-Quarter of the Plate: Lean proteins (e.g., chicken, fish, tofu)

One-Quarter of the Plate: Whole grains or starchy vegetables (e.g., brown rice, quinoa, sweet potatoes)

Adding a serving of fruit and a serving of dairy can complete the meal, ensuring a balanced intake of all macronutrients.

c. Glycemic Index and Load

The glycemic index (GI) measures how quickly a carbohydrate-containing food raises blood sugar levels. Foods with a high GI cause rapid spikes in blood sugar, while foods with a low GI result in a slower, more gradual increase. The glycemic load (GL) takes into account the GI and the carbohydrate content in a serving, providing a more comprehensive picture of a food's impact on blood sugar.

Diabetics should focus on low to moderate GI foods, such as whole grains, legumes, non-starchy vegetables, and most fruits. High GI foods, like white bread, sugary snacks, and processed foods, should be limited.

3. Portion Control

Portion control is critical for managing blood sugar levels and preventing overeating. Consuming large portions, especially of carbohydrate-rich foods, can lead to significant increases in blood sugar levels.

a. Measuring Portions

Using measuring cups, spoons, and a food scale can help accurately measure portions. Understanding standard serving sizes is also essential. For example:

One serving of carbohydrates: 1 slice of bread, 1/3 cup of cooked rice, or 1 small piece of fruit

One serving of protein: 3 ounces of cooked meat, 1 egg, or 1/2 cup of beans

One serving of fats: 1 teaspoon of oil, 1/4 avocado, or 1 ounce of nuts

b. Visual Cues

Visual cues can be helpful for estimating portion sizes when measuring tools are not available. For instance:

1 cup of vegetables: Approximately the size of a fist

3 ounces of meat: The size of a deck of cards

1 teaspoon of oil: About the size of the tip of a thumb

c. Mindful Eating

Mindful eating involves paying attention to hunger and fullness cues, eating slowly, and savoring each bite. This practice can help prevent overeating and promote better digestion.

## 4. Timing of Meals

The timing of meals is another crucial aspect of managing diabetes. Eating at regular intervals helps maintain stable blood sugar levels and prevents extreme highs and lows.

### a. Regular Meal Schedule

Eating three balanced meals a day with snacks in between can help keep blood sugar levels stable. Skipping meals can lead to low blood sugar (hypoglycemia), while overeating at one sitting can cause high blood sugar (hyperglycemia).

### b. Small, Frequent Meals

Some diabetics find that eating smaller, more frequent meals helps maintain more consistent blood sugar levels. This approach can prevent large fluctuations and provide a steady supply of energy throughout the day.

### c. Bedtime Snacks

A small, balanced snack before bedtime can prevent blood sugar levels from dropping too low during the night. Good options include a piece of fruit with a small amount of cheese, a handful of nuts, or a whole-grain cracker with peanut butter.

# 4.2 Creating a 28-Day Meal Plan

Creating a 28-day meal plan tailored for individuals with diabetes involves careful planning and consideration of nutritional needs. This plan should focus on maintaining stable blood sugar levels, providing balanced nutrition, and incorporating the principles of Dr. Barbara O'Neill's approach to diabetes management. Below, we will detail how to construct a 28-day meal plan, including tips for meal preparation and planning.

## Principles of Meal Planning for Diabetes

1. Balancing Macronutrients

Carbohydrates: Choose complex carbohydrates with a low glycemic index (GI) to avoid rapid spikes in blood sugar. Examples include whole grains, legumes, and non-starchy vegetables.

Proteins: Incorporate lean proteins such as chicken, fish, tofu, and legumes. Protein helps in muscle repair and provides satiety.

Fats: Include healthy fats from sources like avocados, nuts, seeds, and olive oil. Healthy fats can improve blood sugar control and heart health.

2. Portion Control and Timing

Portion Sizes: Ensure portion sizes are appropriate to avoid overeating. Using smaller plates and measuring portions can help.

Meal Timing: Eat meals at regular intervals to maintain stable blood sugar levels. Aim for three main meals and 1-2 snacks per day.

## Creating a 28-Day Meal Plan

Week 1:

Day 1:

Breakfast: Oatmeal with Berries and Almonds

Ingredients: Rolled oats, fresh berries (blueberries, strawberries), sliced almonds, a pinch of cinnamon.

Preparation: Cook the oats as per package instructions. Top with berries, almonds, and cinnamon.

Lunch: Grilled Chicken Salad

Ingredients: Grilled chicken breast, mixed greens (spinach, kale, arugula), cherry tomatoes, cucumber, avocado, olive oil, lemon juice.

Preparation: Grill the chicken breast. Toss the mixed greens with cherry tomatoes, cucumber, and avocado. Dress with olive oil and lemon juice.

Dinner: Baked Salmon with Quinoa and Steamed Broccoli

Ingredients: Salmon fillet, quinoa, broccoli, olive oil, garlic, lemon.

Preparation: Bake the salmon with a drizzle of olive oil, minced garlic, and lemon slices. Cook quinoa as per package instructions. Steam the broccoli.

Snack: Greek Yogurt with Nuts

Ingredients: Plain Greek yogurt, mixed nuts (walnuts, almonds, pistachios).

Preparation: Top Greek yogurt with a handful of mixed nuts.

Day 2:

Breakfast: Smoothie with Spinach, Banana, and Chia Seeds

Ingredients: Fresh spinach, banana, chia seeds, unsweetened almond milk.

Preparation: Blend spinach, banana, chia seeds, and almond milk until smooth.

Lunch: Lentil Soup

Ingredients: Lentils, carrots, celery, onion, garlic, vegetable broth, bay leaf.

Preparation: Sauté onions, garlic, carrots, and celery. Add lentils, vegetable broth, and bay leaf. Simmer until lentils are tender.

Dinner: Turkey Stir-Fry with Brown Rice

Ingredients: Ground turkey, mixed vegetables (bell peppers, broccoli, snap peas), brown rice, soy sauce, ginger, garlic.

Preparation: Cook ground turkey with minced garlic and ginger. Add mixed vegetables and stir-fry. Serve over brown rice.

Snack: Apple Slices with Peanut Butter

Ingredients: Apple, natural peanut butter.

Preparation: Slice the apple and dip in peanut butter.

Days 3-7:

Follow a similar structure with varied recipes to include different proteins, vegetables, and whole grains. Ensure a balance of macronutrients and incorporate Dr. Barbara O'Neill's recommended herbs.

Sample Weekly Meal Plan Template:

| Day | Breakfast | Lunch | Dinner | Snack |
|---|---|---|---|---|
| Day 1 | Oatmeal with Berries and Almonds | Grilled Chicken Salad | Baked Salmon with Quinoa and Broccoli | Greek Yogurt with Nuts |
| Day 2 | Smoothie with Spinach, Banana | Lentil Soup | Turkey Stir-Fry with Brown Rice | Apple Slices with Peanut Butter |

Day 3 Avocado Toast with Eggs Chickpea and Vegetable Wrap   Grilled        Shrimp with Zoodles        Cottage Cheese with Berries

Day 4 Greek Yogurt Parfait        Quinoa Salad with Roasted Veggies     Baked Chicken with Sweet Potato        Mixed Nuts

Day 5 Chia Seed Pudding Tuna Salad Lettuce Wrap Beef   and   Vegetable   Kebabs        Hummus with Carrot Sticks

Day 6 Scrambled Tofu with Veggies     Black Bean Soup     Stuffed     Bell     Peppers        Celery with Almond Butter

Day 7 Smoothie Bowl      Turkey and Avocado Salad       Grilled       Fish       with Cauliflower Rice     Edamame

Tips for Meal Preparation and Planning:

Plan Ahead: Take some time each week to plan meals and create a shopping list. This reduces stress and ensures you have all the ingredients on hand.

Batch Cooking: Prepare large batches of meals that can be stored in the refrigerator or freezer for quick and easy meals throughout the week.

Prep Ingredients: Wash and chop vegetables, marinate proteins, and portion out snacks ahead of time to streamline meal preparation.

Use Leftovers: Incorporate leftovers into new meals to minimize food waste and save time. For example, leftover grilled chicken can be used in salads, wraps, or stir-fries.

Stay Flexible: Be open to adjusting the meal plan based on availability of ingredients, seasonal produce, and personal preferences.

Incorporate Herbs: Use Dr. Barbara O'Neill's recommended herbs in your meals. Add cinnamon to oatmeal, include fresh herbs like parsley and cilantro in salads, and use ginger and garlic in stir-fries and soups.

Sample Recipes:

Oatmeal with Berries and Almonds

Ingredients:

1 cup rolled oats

1 cup fresh berries (blueberries, strawberries)

1/4 cup sliced almonds

1/2 tsp cinnamon

2 cups water or unsweetened almond milk

Preparation:

In a pot, bring water or almond milk to a boil.

Add rolled oats and reduce heat to a simmer. Cook for about 5-7 minutes, stirring occasionally.

Once the oats are cooked, remove from heat and stir in cinnamon.

Top with fresh berries and sliced almonds before serving.

Grilled Chicken Salad

Ingredients:

1 grilled chicken breast

4 cups mixed greens (spinach, kale, arugula)

1 cup cherry tomatoes, halved

1 cucumber, sliced

1 avocado, sliced

2 tbsp olive oil

1 tbsp lemon juice

Salt and pepper to taste

Preparation:

Grill the chicken breast until fully cooked and set aside to cool.

In a large bowl, combine mixed greens, cherry tomatoes, cucumber, and avocado.

Slice the grilled chicken and add to the salad.

Drizzle with olive oil and lemon juice, and season with salt and pepper. Toss to combine and serve.

Baked Salmon with Quinoa and Steamed Broccoli

Ingredients:

1 salmon fillet

1 cup quinoa

2 cups broccoli florets

2 tbsp olive oil

2 cloves garlic, minced

1 lemon, sliced

Salt and pepper to taste

Preparation:

Preheat the oven to 375°F (190°C).

Place the salmon fillet on a baking sheet lined with parchment paper. Drizzle with olive oil, sprinkle with minced garlic, and top with lemon slices. Season with salt and pepper.

Bake for 15-20 minutes, until the salmon is fully cooked.

Meanwhile, rinse quinoa under cold water. In a pot, combine quinoa with 2 cups of water. Bring to a boil, then reduce heat to a simmer and cook for about 15 minutes, until water is absorbed.

Steam broccoli florets until tender.

Serve the baked salmon over a bed of quinoa with steamed broccoli on the side.

# 4.3: Sample 28-Day Meal Plan

Creating a comprehensive 28-day meal plan tailored to managing diabetes involves balancing nutrient-rich foods that help maintain stable blood sugar levels. This meal plan is designed to be easy to follow, delicious, and nutritionally balanced, incorporating Dr. Barbara O'Neill's principles and herbal remedies.

Week 1: Breakfast, Lunch, Dinner, and Snacks

Day 1

Breakfast: Spinach and Mushroom Omelet

Ingredients:

2 eggs

1 cup fresh spinach

1/2 cup mushrooms, sliced

1/4 cup onion, diced

1 tablespoon olive oil

Salt and pepper to taste

Instructions:

Heat olive oil in a pan over medium heat.

Add onions and mushrooms, sauté until soft.

Add spinach and cook until wilted.

Beat eggs in a bowl, then pour into the pan.

Cook until eggs are set, fold and serve.

Lunch: Quinoa Salad with Chickpeas and Herbs

Ingredients:

1 cup cooked quinoa

1/2 cup canned chickpeas, drained and rinsed

1/2 cucumber, diced

1/4 cup red bell pepper, diced

1/4 cup fresh parsley, chopped

1/4 cup feta cheese, crumbled

2 tablespoons olive oil

1 tablespoon lemon juice

Salt and pepper to taste

Instructions:

In a large bowl, combine quinoa, chickpeas, cucumber, bell pepper, and parsley.

In a small bowl, whisk together olive oil, lemon juice, salt, and pepper.

Pour dressing over salad, toss to combine.

Sprinkle with feta cheese before serving.

Dinner: Baked Salmon with Asparagus


Ingredients:

1 salmon fillet

1 bunch asparagus, trimmed

2 tablespoons olive oil

1 tablespoon fresh lemon juice

2 cloves garlic, minced

Salt and pepper to taste

Instructions:

Preheat oven to 375°F (190°C).

Place salmon and asparagus on a baking sheet.

Drizzle with olive oil, lemon juice, and minced garlic.

Season with salt and pepper.

Bake for 20 minutes or until salmon is cooked through.

Snack: Apple Slices with Almond Butter

Ingredients:

1 apple, sliced

2 tablespoons almond butter

Instructions:

Slice the apple and spread almond butter on each slice.

Enjoy as a healthy snack.

Day 2

Breakfast: Greek Yogurt with Berries and Chia Seeds

Ingredients:

1 cup Greek yogurt

1/2 cup mixed berries (strawberries, blueberries, raspberries)

1 tablespoon chia seeds

Instructions:

Place Greek yogurt in a bowl.

Top with mixed berries and chia seeds.

Stir gently and serve.

Lunch: Lentil Soup with Fresh Herbs

Ingredients:

1 cup lentils, rinsed

1 carrot, diced

1 celery stalk, diced

1 onion, chopped

2 cloves garlic, minced

4 cups vegetable broth

1 tablespoon olive oil

1 bay leaf

1/4 cup fresh parsley, chopped

Salt and pepper to taste

Instructions:

Heat olive oil in a large pot over medium heat.

Add onion, carrot, and celery, cook until soft.

Add garlic, cook for another minute.

Add lentils, vegetable broth, and bay leaf.

Bring to a boil, then reduce heat and simmer for 30 minutes.

Remove bay leaf, season with salt, pepper, and parsley.

Dinner: Grilled Chicken with Steamed Broccoli

Ingredients:

1 chicken breast

1 bunch broccoli, cut into florets

1 tablespoon olive oil

1 teaspoon garlic powder

Salt and pepper to taste

Instructions:

Preheat grill to medium-high heat.

Season chicken breast with olive oil, garlic powder, salt, and pepper.

Grill chicken for 6-7 minutes on each side until cooked through.

Steam broccoli until tender, about 5 minutes.

Snack: Celery Sticks with Hummus

Ingredients:

4 celery sticks, cut into pieces

1/4 cup hummus

Instructions:

Cut celery sticks into pieces.

Serve with hummus for dipping.

Day 3

Breakfast: Oatmeal with Nuts and Berries

Ingredients:

1/2 cup rolled oats

1 cup water or almond milk

1/4 cup mixed nuts (almonds, walnuts, pecans)

1/4 cup mixed berries (blueberries, raspberries, strawberries)

1 tablespoon flax seeds

Instructions:

In a pot, bring water or almond milk to a boil.

Add oats and cook for 5-7 minutes, stirring occasionally.

Top with nuts, berries, and flax seeds before serving.

Lunch: Turkey and Avocado Wrap

Ingredients:

1 whole grain tortilla

3 slices of turkey breast

1/2 avocado, sliced

1/4 cup shredded lettuce

1/4 cup diced tomatoes

1 tablespoon mustard or light mayonnaise

Instructions:

Lay the tortilla flat and spread mustard or mayonnaise.

Layer turkey, avocado, lettuce, and tomatoes.

Roll up the tortilla and slice in half.

Dinner: Stuffed Bell Peppers

Ingredients:

2 bell peppers, halved and seeded

1/2 cup cooked quinoa

1/2 cup black beans, drained and rinsed

1/4 cup corn kernels

1/4 cup diced tomatoes

1/4 cup shredded cheese (optional)

1 tablespoon olive oil

1 teaspoon cumin

Salt and pepper to taste

Instructions:

Preheat oven to 375°F (190°C).

In a bowl, mix quinoa, black beans, corn, tomatoes, olive oil, cumin, salt, and pepper.

Stuff the bell peppers with the mixture.

Place in a baking dish and bake for 30 minutes.

Top with cheese, if using, and bake for another 5 minutes.

Snack: Mixed Nuts and Seeds

Ingredients:

1/4 cup mixed nuts (almonds, walnuts, cashews)

1/4 cup mixed seeds (pumpkin, sunflower, chia)

Instructions:

Combine nuts and seeds in a small bowl.

Enjoy as a snack.

Day 4

Breakfast: Smoothie with Spinach and Protein

Ingredients:

1 cup spinach

1 banana

1/2 cup Greek yogurt

1 tablespoon chia seeds

1 cup almond milk

Instructions:

Place all ingredients in a blender.

Blend until smooth and creamy.

Pour into a glass and serve.

Lunch: Grilled Vegetable and Hummus Sandwich

Ingredients:

2 slices whole grain bread

1/4 cup hummus

1/4 cup grilled zucchini

1/4 cup grilled eggplant

1/4 cup roasted red peppers

Instructions:

Spread hummus on each slice of bread.

Layer grilled vegetables on one slice.

Top with the other slice of bread and serve.

Dinner: Beef Stir-Fry with Vegetables

Ingredients:

1 cup sliced beef

1 cup broccoli florets

1 bell pepper, sliced

1/2 cup snow peas

2 tablespoons soy sauce (low sodium)

1 tablespoon olive oil

1 teaspoon ginger, grated

2 cloves garlic, minced

Instructions:

Heat olive oil in a large pan over medium-high heat.

Add garlic and ginger, sauté for 1 minute.

Add beef and cook until browned.

Add vegetables and soy sauce, cook until tender.

Serve over brown rice or quinoa.

Snack: Carrot Sticks with Guacamole

Ingredients:

2 carrots, cut into sticks

1/4 cup guacamole

Instructions:

Cut carrots into sticks.

Serve with guacamole for dipping.

Day 5

Breakfast: Chia Pudding with Almonds and Blueberries

Ingredients:

1/4 cup chia seeds

1 cup almond milk

1/2 cup blueberries

1/4 cup sliced almonds

Instructions:

In a bowl, combine chia seeds and almond milk.

Stir well and refrigerate overnight.

In the morning, top with blueberries and almonds.

Lunch: Chicken Caesar Salad

Ingredients:

2 cups romaine lettuce, chopped

1 grilled chicken breast, sliced

1/4 cup grated Parmesan cheese

1/4 cup croutons (optional)

2 tablespoons Caesar dressing

Instructions:

In a large bowl, combine lettuce, chicken, Parmesan, and croutons.

Drizzle with Caesar dressing and toss to coat.

Dinner: Shrimp Tacos with Avocado Salsa

Ingredients:

1/2 pound shrimp, peeled and deveined

1 tablespoon olive oil

1 teaspoon chili powder

1 avocado, diced

1/4 cup diced red onion

1/4 cup chopped cilantro

1 tablespoon lime juice

Corn tortillas

Instructions:

In a bowl, toss shrimp with olive oil and chili powder.

Cook shrimp in a pan over medium heat until pink and opaque.

In another bowl, combine avocado, red onion, cilantro, and lime juice.

Serve shrimp in corn tortillas topped with avocado salsa.

Snack: Greek Yogurt with Walnuts


Ingredients:

1 cup Greek yogurt

1/4 cup chopped walnuts

Instructions:

Place Greek yogurt in a bowl.

Top with chopped walnuts.

Day 6


Breakfast: Avocado Toast with Poached Egg

Ingredients:

1 slice whole grain bread

1/2 avocado, mashed

1 egg

1 tablespoon vinegar

Salt and pepper to taste

Instructions:

Toast the bread.

Spread mashed avocado on the toast.

Bring a pot of water to a simmer, add vinegar.

Crack egg into a small bowl, gently slide into the water.

Poach for 3-4 minutes, remove with a slotted spoon.

Place poached egg on avocado toast, season with salt and pepper.

Lunch: Tuna Salad Lettuce Wraps


Ingredients:

1 can tuna, drained

2 tablespoons plain Greek yogurt

1 tablespoon Dijon mustard

1 celery stalk, diced

1/4 cup diced red onion

1 tablespoon chopped dill

Large lettuce leaves

Instructions:

In a bowl, combine tuna, Greek yogurt, mustard, celery, onion, and dill.

Spoon mixture onto large lettuce leaves and roll up.

Dinner: Eggplant Parmesan

Ingredients:

1 large eggplant, sliced

1 cup marinara sauce

1/2 cup grated Parmesan cheese

1/2 cup mozzarella cheese, shredded

1 tablespoon olive oil

Salt and pepper to taste

Instructions:

Preheat oven to 375°F (190°C).

Brush eggplant slices with olive oil, season with salt and pepper.

Grill eggplant slices until tender.

Layer eggplant slices, marinara sauce, and cheeses in a baking dish.

Bake for 20 minutes or until cheese is melted and bubbly.

Snack: Bell Pepper Slices with Cream Cheese

Ingredients:

1 bell pepper, sliced

2 tablespoons cream cheese

Instructions:

Slice the bell pepper into strips.

Serve with cream cheese for dipping.

Day 7

Breakfast: Berry Smoothie Bowl

Ingredients:

1 cup mixed berries

1/2 cup Greek yogurt

1/2 cup almond milk

1 tablespoon chia seeds

1/4 cup granola

Instructions:

Blend berries, Greek yogurt, and almond milk until smooth.

Pour into a bowl and top with chia seeds and granola.

Lunch: Black Bean and Corn Salad

Ingredients:

1 can black beans, drained and rinsed

1 cup corn kernels

1/2 red bell pepper, diced

1/4 cup chopped cilantro

1 tablespoon olive oil

1 tablespoon lime juice

Salt and pepper to taste

Instructions:

In a bowl, combine black beans, corn, bell pepper, and cilantro.

Drizzle with olive oil and lime juice, season with salt and pepper.

Toss to combine.

Dinner: Zucchini Noodles with Pesto

Ingredients:

2 large zucchinis, spiralized

1/4 cup basil pesto

1/4 cup cherry tomatoes, halved

2 tablespoons grated Parmesan cheese

Instructions:

In a pan, sauté zucchini noodles for 2-3 minutes until tender.

Add pesto and cherry tomatoes, toss to combine.

Serve with grated Parmesan cheese on top.

Snack: Cottage Cheese with Pineapple

Ingredients:

1 cup cottage cheese

1/2 cup pineapple chunks

Instructions:

Place cottage cheese in a bowl.

Top with pineapple chunks and serve.

# 4.4 Adapting the Meal Plan to Individual Needs

Creating a meal plan that works for everyone can be challenging due to individual differences in health status, dietary preferences, and lifestyle. This section will help you adapt the 28-day meal plan to suit your unique needs, ensuring it is both enjoyable and effective for managing diabetes. Here, we will explore modifications for specific dietary restrictions, adjustments based on activity levels, and personal preferences, providing practical tips and examples.

# Understanding Individual Dietary Needs

Adapting a meal plan begins with understanding your specific dietary needs. People with diabetes often have varying requirements based on factors such as age, weight, activity level, and any additional health conditions. Here are key considerations:

Age: Nutritional needs change with age. For instance, older adults may require more calcium and vitamin D for bone health, while younger individuals might need higher protein intake for muscle maintenance.

Weight: Those aiming for weight loss might need a reduced-calorie plan, while others seeking to maintain or gain weight may require more calories.

Activity Level: Active individuals typically need more carbohydrates and overall calories compared to those with a sedentary lifestyle.

Health Conditions: Conditions such as hypertension, kidney disease, or gluten intolerance necessitate specific dietary adjustments.

Modifications for Specific Dietary Restrictions

Gluten-Free Diet

For those with celiac disease or gluten sensitivity, it's essential to avoid gluten-containing foods. Here are some swaps and recipe adjustments:

Breakfast: Substitute regular pancakes with gluten-free pancakes made from almond flour or coconut flour. Ensure oats are certified gluten-free.

Lunch and Dinner: Use gluten-free grains such as quinoa, brown rice, or gluten-free pasta. Replace bread with gluten-free bread or lettuce wraps.

Snacks: Opt for gluten-free crackers, rice cakes, or homemade snacks using gluten-free ingredients.

Example Recipe: Gluten-Free Pancakes

Ingredients:

1 cup almond flour

2 eggs

1/4 cup unsweetened almond milk

1 tsp baking powder

1 tsp vanilla extract

1/2 tsp cinnamon

Instructions:

In a bowl, whisk together all ingredients until smooth.

Heat a non-stick skillet over medium heat and lightly grease it with oil.

Pour batter onto the skillet, forming small pancakes.

Cook until bubbles form on the surface, then flip and cook until golden brown.

Serve with fresh berries and a drizzle of sugar-free syrup.

Vegetarian/Vegan Diet

For those following a vegetarian or vegan diet, it's crucial to ensure adequate protein intake. Here are some tips:

Protein Sources: Include plant-based proteins like beans, lentils, tofu, tempeh, and quinoa.

Meal Adjustments: Replace meat in recipes with these protein sources. For example, use black beans in chili or tofu in stir-fries.

Dairy Alternatives: Use almond milk, coconut milk, or soy milk instead of dairy milk. Substitute cheese with vegan cheese alternatives.

Example Recipe: Vegan Quinoa Salad

Ingredients:

1 cup cooked quinoa

1 cup cherry tomatoes, halved

1 cucumber, diced

1/2 red onion, finely chopped

1 cup chickpeas, drained and rinsed

1/4 cup fresh parsley, chopped

Juice of 1 lemon

2 tbsp olive oil

Salt and pepper to taste

Instructions:

In a large bowl, combine quinoa, cherry tomatoes, cucumber, red onion, chickpeas, and parsley.

In a small bowl, whisk together lemon juice, olive oil, salt, and pepper.

Pour the dressing over the salad and toss to combine.

Serve chilled.

Low-Sodium Diet

For individuals with hypertension or other conditions requiring a low-sodium diet, reducing salt intake is vital. Here are some strategies:

Seasoning Alternatives: Use herbs, spices, lemon juice, and vinegar to add flavor without salt.

Avoid Processed Foods: Processed foods often contain high sodium levels. Opt for fresh, whole foods.

**Read Labels:** Always check nutrition labels for sodium content and choose low-sodium options.

Example Recipe: Herb-Roasted Chicken

Ingredients:

4 boneless, skinless chicken breasts

2 tbsp olive oil

1 tsp garlic powder

1 tsp dried thyme

1 tsp dried rosemary

1 tsp paprika

1 lemon, sliced

Freshly ground black pepper to taste

Instructions:

Preheat the oven to 375°F (190°C).

In a small bowl, mix olive oil, garlic powder, thyme, rosemary, and paprika.

Rub the mixture over the chicken breasts.

Place chicken in a baking dish, top with lemon slices, and sprinkle with black pepper.

Bake for 25-30 minutes or until the chicken is cooked through.

Serve with a side of steamed vegetables.

## Adjusting for Activity Levels

### High Activity Levels

For those with a high activity level, it's important to fuel the body adequately:

Carbohydrate Intake: Increase carbohydrate intake to support energy needs. Opt for whole grains, fruits, and starchy vegetables.

Protein for Recovery: Ensure sufficient protein intake to aid muscle recovery and growth. Include protein-rich snacks post-workout, such as a protein smoothie or a handful of nuts.

### Example Recipe: Post-Workout Smoothie

Ingredients:

1 banana

1 cup unsweetened almond milk

1 tbsp almond butter

1 scoop plant-based protein powder

1 tsp honey (optional)

Ice cubes

Instructions:

Combine all ingredients in a blender.

Blend until smooth.

Pour into a glass and enjoy.

Low Activity Levels

For those with a sedentary lifestyle, it's essential to manage calorie intake to prevent weight gain:

Portion Control: Focus on portion control and avoid overeating.

Low-Calorie Foods: Emphasize low-calorie, nutrient-dense foods like vegetables, lean proteins, and whole grains.

Example Recipe: Zucchini Noodles with Pesto

Ingredients:

2 large zucchinis, spiralized

1 cup cherry tomatoes, halved

1/4 cup homemade or store-bought pesto

2 tbsp pine nuts

Grated Parmesan cheese (optional)

Instructions:

In a large skillet, sauté zucchini noodles over medium heat for 3-4 minutes until tender.

Add cherry tomatoes and cook for an additional 2 minutes.

Remove from heat and toss with pesto.

Top with pine nuts and Parmesan cheese, if desired.

Serve immediately.

Adjusting for Personal Preferences

Flavor Preferences

Adapting meals to suit flavor preferences ensures that you enjoy your diet and stick with it:

Spicy Foods: Add spices like chili powder, cayenne pepper, or hot sauce to meals.

Mild Foods: Opt for herbs like basil, parsley, and thyme for a milder flavor profile.

Example Recipe: Spicy Black Bean Tacos

Ingredients:

1 can black beans, drained and rinsed

1 tsp chili powder

1/2 tsp cumin

1/2 tsp paprika

8 small corn tortillas

1 avocado, sliced

1/2 red onion, diced

Fresh cilantro, chopped

Lime wedges

Instructions:

In a skillet, heat black beans over medium heat. Add chili powder, cumin, and paprika, stirring to combine.

Cook until beans are heated through.

Warm tortillas in a separate skillet or microwave.

Fill tortillas with black beans, avocado slices, red onion, and cilantro.

Serve with lime wedges.

Texture Preferences

Some people prefer certain textures in their meals, such as crunchy or creamy:

Crunchy: Include raw vegetables, nuts, and seeds for added crunch.

Creamy: Use ingredients like avocado, Greek yogurt, or hummus for a creamy texture.

Example Recipe: Crunchy Veggie Wraps

Ingredients:

4 large whole wheat tortillas

1 cup hummus

1 cup shredded carrots

1 cucumber, julienned

1 bell pepper, sliced

1/4 cup sunflower seeds

Fresh spinach leaves

Instructions:

Spread hummus evenly over each tortilla.

Layer with shredded carrots, cucumber, bell pepper, sunflower seeds, and spinach leaves.

Roll up tightly and slice in half.

Serve immediately or wrap in foil for a portable meal.

# Chapter 5: 365 Days of Mouthwatering Recipes

## 5.1: Breakfast Recipes

Breakfast is often called the most important meal of the day, especially for individuals managing diabetes. A balanced breakfast can help stabilize blood sugar levels, provide essential nutrients, and set a positive tone for the day. In this subchapter, we present a collection of delicious, nutritious, and diabetes-friendly breakfast recipes. Each recipe is designed to be easy to prepare, packed with nutrients, and mindful of carbohydrate content.

# Smoothies and Shakes

1. Berry Spinach Smoothie

Ingredients:

1 cup fresh spinach

1/2 cup frozen mixed berries (blueberries, strawberries, raspberries)

1/2 cup unsweetened almond milk

1/2 cup plain Greek yogurt

1 tablespoon chia seeds

1 teaspoon honey (optional)

1/2 teaspoon vanilla extract

Instructions:

Combine all ingredients in a blender.

Blend until smooth and creamy.

Pour into a glass and enjoy immediately.

Benefits:

This smoothie is high in fiber, antioxidants, and protein. The berries add a natural sweetness while the spinach provides essential vitamins and minerals. Greek yogurt and chia seeds boost the protein content, making this smoothie a satisfying and balanced breakfast option.

## 2. Peanut Butter Banana Smoothie

Ingredients:

1 medium banana

1 tablespoon natural peanut butter

1/2 cup unsweetened almond milk

1/2 cup plain Greek yogurt

1 tablespoon flax seeds

Ice cubes (optional)

Instructions:

Add all ingredients to a blender.

Blend until smooth.

Pour into a glass and enjoy immediately.

Benefits:

This smoothie offers a good balance of protein, healthy fats, and carbohydrates. Bananas provide natural sweetness and potassium, while peanut butter and flax seeds add healthy fats and protein.

Omelets and Scrambles

1. Veggie-Packed Omelet

Ingredients:

2 large eggs

1/4 cup chopped bell peppers (any color)

1/4 cup chopped onions

1/4 cup chopped tomatoes

1/4 cup chopped spinach

1/4 cup shredded low-fat cheese

1 tablespoon olive oil

Salt and pepper to taste

Instructions:

Heat olive oil in a non-stick skillet over medium heat.

Add bell peppers, onions, and tomatoes. Sauté until vegetables are tender.

Add spinach and cook until wilted.

In a bowl, whisk eggs with a pinch of salt and pepper.

Pour eggs over the sautéed vegetables in the skillet.

Cook until eggs are set, then sprinkle cheese on top.

Fold the omelet in half and cook for another minute until cheese is melted.

Serve hot.

Benefits:

This omelet is loaded with vegetables, providing fiber, vitamins, and minerals. The eggs offer high-quality protein, and the cheese adds a touch of calcium and flavor without too much fat.

2. Tofu Scramble

Ingredients:

1 block firm tofu, drained and crumbled

1/4 cup chopped onions

1/4 cup chopped bell peppers

1/4 cup chopped tomatoes

1/4 cup chopped spinach

1 tablespoon olive oil

1/2 teaspoon turmeric

1/2 teaspoon cumin

Salt and pepper to taste

Instructions:

Heat olive oil in a skillet over medium heat.

Add onions and bell peppers, and sauté until tender.

Add crumbled tofu, turmeric, and cumin. Stir well to coat the tofu with spices.

Add tomatoes and spinach, cooking until spinach is wilted.

Season with salt and pepper to taste.

Serve hot.

Benefits:

Tofu is a great source of plant-based protein and can mimic the texture of scrambled eggs. The vegetables add essential nutrients and fiber, while turmeric provides anti-inflammatory benefits.

## Diabetic-Friendly Pancakes and Waffles

1. Almond Flour Pancakes

Ingredients:

1 cup almond flour

2 large eggs

1/4 cup unsweetened almond milk

1 teaspoon baking powder

1/2 teaspoon vanilla extract

1/4 teaspoon salt

Cooking spray or butter for the pan

Instructions:

In a bowl, whisk together almond flour, baking powder, and salt.

In another bowl, beat the eggs, then add almond milk and vanilla extract.

Combine the wet and dry ingredients, stirring until smooth.

Heat a non-stick skillet over medium heat and coat with cooking spray or butter.

Pour small amounts of batter onto the skillet to form pancakes.

Cook until bubbles form on the surface, then flip and cook until golden brown.

Serve warm with a sugar-free syrup or fresh berries.

Benefits:

Almond flour is low in carbohydrates and high in protein and healthy fats. These pancakes are a delicious and satisfying low-carb breakfast option.

## 2. Whole Wheat Waffles

Ingredients:

1 cup whole wheat flour

1 teaspoon baking powder

1/4 teaspoon salt

1 tablespoon stevia or other sugar substitute

1 large egg

1 cup unsweetened almond milk

2 tablespoons melted coconut oil

1/2 teaspoon vanilla extract

Instructions:

Preheat the waffle iron.

In a large bowl, whisk together whole wheat flour, baking powder, salt, and stevia.

In another bowl, beat the egg and then add almond milk, melted coconut oil, and vanilla extract.

Combine wet and dry ingredients, stirring until smooth.

Pour batter into the preheated waffle iron and cook according to the manufacturer's instructions.

Serve warm with a sugar-free syrup or fresh fruit.

Benefits:

Whole wheat flour adds fiber and nutrients to these waffles, making them a healthier choice compared to traditional white flour waffles. They are filling and can help maintain steady blood sugar levels.

Pictures

Since including actual pictures isn't possible here, consider these visual descriptions:

Berry Spinach Smoothie: A vibrant green smoothie with specks of colorful berries, served in a clear glass.

Peanut Butter Banana Smoothie: A creamy, light beige smoothie with a sprinkle of flax seeds on top, served in a mason jar.

Veggie-Packed Omelet: A golden omelet filled with colorful sautéed vegetables and melted cheese, folded neatly on a white plate.

Tofu Scramble: A bright yellow scramble mixed with red and green vegetables, served in a rustic bowl.

Almond Flour Pancakes: A stack of fluffy, golden-brown pancakes, topped with fresh berries and a drizzle of syrup.

Whole Wheat Waffles: Crispy, golden waffles with a grid pattern, topped with a dollop of Greek yogurt and a handful of fresh berries.

# 5.2: Lunch Recipes

Lunch is a crucial meal for those managing diabetes, providing an opportunity to balance blood sugar levels and maintain energy throughout the afternoon. Here, we present a variety of lunch recipes that are not only diabetic-friendly but also delicious and satisfying. These recipes are designed to be easy to prepare, using readily available ingredients. Each recipe is constructed with a focus on balancing carbohydrates, proteins, and healthy fats to help stabilize blood sugar levels.

Salad Recipes

1. Quinoa and Kale Salad

Ingredients:

1 cup quinoa, rinsed

2 cups water

2 cups chopped kale

1 cup cherry tomatoes, halved

1/2 cup cucumber, diced

1/4 cup red onion, finely chopped

1/4 cup crumbled feta cheese

2 tablespoons olive oil

2 tablespoons lemon juice

Salt and pepper to taste

Instructions:


In a medium saucepan, bring quinoa and water to a boil. Reduce heat, cover, and simmer for 15 minutes or until quinoa is tender and water is absorbed. Fluff with a fork and let cool.

In a large bowl, combine kale, cherry tomatoes, cucumber, red onion, and feta cheese.

Add cooked quinoa to the salad mixture.

In a small bowl, whisk together olive oil, lemon juice, salt, and pepper.

Pour the dressing over the salad and toss to combine.

Serve immediately or refrigerate for later.

Nutritional Information:

Calories: 250 per serving

Carbohydrates: 35g

Protein: 8g

Fat: 10g

Photo:

## 2. Grilled Chicken Caesar Salad

Ingredients:

2 boneless, skinless chicken breasts

1 tablespoon olive oil

Salt and pepper to taste

6 cups Romaine lettuce, chopped

1/4 cup grated Parmesan cheese

1/2 cup cherry tomatoes, halved

1/4 cup Caesar dressing (preferably low-fat)

Instructions:

Preheat the grill to medium-high heat.

Brush chicken breasts with olive oil and season with salt and pepper.

Grill chicken for 6-7 minutes on each side or until fully cooked. Let rest for 5 minutes before slicing.

In a large bowl, combine Romaine lettuce, Parmesan cheese, and cherry tomatoes.

Slice the grilled chicken and add it to the salad.

Drizzle Caesar dressing over the top and toss to combine.

Serve immediately.

Nutritional Information:

Calories: 320 per serving

Carbohydrates: 12g

Protein: 36g

Fat: 15g

Photo:

## 3. Lentil and Spinach Salad

Ingredients:

1 cup lentils, rinsed and drained

3 cups water

3 cups baby spinach

1/2 cup cherry tomatoes, halved

1/4 cup red bell pepper, diced

1/4 cup red onion, finely chopped

2 tablespoons olive oil

2 tablespoons balsamic vinegar

Salt and pepper to taste

Instructions:

In a medium saucepan, bring lentils and water to a boil. Reduce heat, cover, and simmer for 20-25 minutes or until lentils are tender. Drain and let cool.

In a large bowl, combine baby spinach, cherry tomatoes, red bell pepper, and red onion.

Add cooked lentils to the salad mixture.

In a small bowl, whisk together olive oil, balsamic vinegar, salt, and pepper.

Pour the dressing over the salad and toss to combine.

Serve immediately or refrigerate for later.

Nutritional Information:


Calories: 220 per serving

Carbohydrates: 30g

Protein: 12g

Fat: 7g

Photo:

Soup Recipes

1. Tomato Basil Soup

Ingredients:

2 tablespoons olive oil

1 medium onion, chopped

2 cloves garlic, minced

1 (28-ounce) can crushed tomatoes

2 cups vegetable broth

1/4 cup fresh basil, chopped

Salt and pepper to taste

1/4 cup heavy cream (optional)

Instructions:

In a large pot, heat olive oil over medium heat. Add onion and garlic, sauté until translucent.

Add crushed tomatoes and vegetable broth. Bring to a boil, then reduce heat and simmer for 20 minutes.

Stir in fresh basil, salt, and pepper.

For a creamy soup, stir in heavy cream just before serving.

Use an immersion blender to puree the soup until smooth, or leave it chunky if preferred.

Serve hot.

Nutritional Information:

Calories: 150 per serving

Carbohydrates: 18g

Protein: 3g

Fat: 8g

Photo:

## 2. Chicken and Vegetable Soup

Ingredients:

1 tablespoon olive oil

1 medium onion, chopped

2 cloves garlic, minced

2 medium carrots, sliced

2 celery stalks, sliced

1 zucchini, diced

6 cups chicken broth

2 cups cooked, shredded chicken breast

1 teaspoon dried thyme

1 teaspoon dried oregano

Salt and pepper to taste

Instructions:

In a large pot, heat olive oil over medium heat. Add onion and garlic, sauté until translucent.

Add carrots, celery, and zucchini, sauté for 5 minutes.

Pour in chicken broth and bring to a boil.

Reduce heat and add shredded chicken, thyme, oregano, salt, and pepper.

Simmer for 20 minutes, until vegetables are tender.

Serve hot.

Nutritional Information:

Calories: 200 per serving

Carbohydrates: 12g

Protein: 20g

Fat: 7g

Photo:

## 3. Lentil and Sweet Potato Soup

Ingredients:

1 tablespoon olive oil

1 medium onion, chopped

2 cloves garlic, minced

1 large sweet potato, peeled and diced

1 cup lentils, rinsed

4 cups vegetable broth

1 teaspoon ground cumin

1 teaspoon ground coriander

Salt and pepper to taste

Instructions:

In a large pot, heat olive oil over medium heat. Add onion and garlic, sauté until translucent.

Add sweet potato and lentils, sauté for 5 minutes.

Pour in vegetable broth, cumin, coriander, salt, and pepper. Bring to a boil.

Reduce heat and simmer for 30 minutes, until sweet potato and lentils are tender.

Use an immersion blender to puree the soup until smooth, or leave it chunky if preferred.

Serve hot.

Nutritional Information:

Calories: 250 per serving

Carbohydrates: 45g

Protein: 10g

Fat: 4g

Photo:

Sandwich and Wrap Recipes

1. Turkey and Avocado Wrap

Ingredients:

1 whole wheat tortilla

3 slices deli turkey breast

1/4 avocado, sliced

1/4 cup baby spinach

1/4 cup shredded carrots

2 tablespoons hummus

Instructions:

Lay the tortilla flat and spread hummus evenly over it.

Layer turkey slices, avocado, baby spinach, and shredded carrots on top.

Roll up the tortilla tightly and slice in half.

Serve immediately.

Nutritional Information:

Calories: 300 per serving

Carbohydrates: 30g

Protein: 20g

Fat: 12g

Photo:

2. Mediterranean Veggie Sandwich

Ingredients:

2 slices whole grain bread

2 tablespoons hummus

1/4 cup cucumber slices

1/4 cup roasted red pepper strips

1/4 cup crumbled feta cheese

1/4 cup baby spinach

Instructions:

Spread hummus on one slice of bread.

Layer cucumber slices, roasted red pepper strips, feta cheese, and baby spinach.

Top with the second slice of bread.

Cut in half and serve immediately.

Nutritional Information:

Calories: 280 per serving

Carbohydrates: 35g

Protein: 10g

Fat: 12g

Photo:

## 3. Tuna Salad Lettuce Wraps

Ingredients:

1 can (5 ounces) tuna, drained

2 tablespoons Greek yogurt

1 tablespoon Dijon mustard

1 tablespoon dill relish

1/4 cup diced celery

1/4 cup diced red onion

Salt and pepper to taste

4 large lettuce leaves

Instructions:

In a bowl, combine tuna, Greek yogurt, Dijon mustard, dill relish, celery, red onion, salt, and pepper. Mix well.

Spoon the tuna mixture onto the center of each lettuce leaf.

Roll up the lettuce leaves and secure with toothpicks if necessary.

Serve immediately.

Nutritional Information:

Calories: 150 per serving

Carbohydrates: 5g

Protein: 20g

Fat: 5g

# Chapter 5.3: Dinner Recipes

Dinner is an important meal for individuals managing diabetes, as it can significantly impact overnight blood sugar levels and overall health. The following recipes are designed to be both delicious and diabetes-friendly, ensuring balanced nutrition without compromising on taste. Each recipe emphasizes low glycemic index ingredients, balanced macronutrients, and portion control to help manage blood sugar levels effectively.

Main Courses with Meat and Fish

Grilled Lemon Herb Chicken

Ingredients:

4 boneless, skinless chicken breasts

1/4 cup olive oil

Juice of 2 lemons

3 cloves garlic, minced

2 teaspoons dried oregano

1 teaspoon dried thyme

Salt and pepper to taste

Fresh parsley for garnish

Instructions:

In a large bowl, whisk together olive oil, lemon juice, garlic, oregano, thyme, salt, and pepper.

Add the chicken breasts to the marinade, ensuring they are well coated. Cover and refrigerate for at least 30 minutes, or up to 2 hours.

Preheat the grill to medium-high heat. Grill the chicken for 6-7 minutes on each side, or until fully cooked.

Garnish with fresh parsley and serve with a side of steamed vegetables or a salad.

Baked Salmon with Dill and Lemon

Ingredients:

4 salmon fillets

2 tablespoons olive oil

Juice and zest of 1 lemon

2 tablespoons fresh dill, chopped

2 cloves garlic, minced

Salt and pepper to taste

Lemon slices for garnish

Instructions:

Preheat the oven to 375°F (190°C). Line a baking sheet with parchment paper.

In a small bowl, mix olive oil, lemon juice, lemon zest, dill, garlic, salt, and pepper.

Place the salmon fillets on the prepared baking sheet. Brush the lemon-dill mixture evenly over the fillets.

Bake for 15-20 minutes, or until the salmon is opaque and flakes easily with a fork.

Garnish with lemon slices and serve with a quinoa salad or roasted vegetables.

Vegetarian and Vegan Options

Stuffed Bell Peppers

Ingredients:

4 large bell peppers (any color), tops cut off and seeds removed

1 cup cooked quinoa

1 can black beans, drained and rinsed

1 cup corn kernels (fresh or frozen)

1 cup diced tomatoes

1 small onion, finely chopped

2 cloves garlic, minced

1 teaspoon cumin

1 teaspoon chili powder

Salt and pepper to taste

1/4 cup chopped fresh cilantro

1/2 cup shredded cheese (optional, for non-vegans)

Instructions:

Preheat the oven to 375°F (190°C). Lightly grease a baking dish.

In a large bowl, combine quinoa, black beans, corn, tomatoes, onion, garlic, cumin, chili powder, salt, and pepper.

Stuff the bell peppers with the quinoa mixture, packing it firmly.

Place the stuffed peppers in the prepared baking dish. Cover with foil and bake for 30 minutes.

Remove the foil and sprinkle with cheese (if using). Bake for an additional 10 minutes, or until the peppers are tender.

Garnish with fresh cilantro and serve with a green salad.

Lentil and Vegetable Stir-Fry

Ingredients:

1 cup dried lentils, rinsed and drained

2 tablespoons olive oil

1 onion, sliced

2 cloves garlic, minced

1 bell pepper, sliced

1 zucchini, sliced

1 carrot, julienned

1 cup broccoli florets

3 tablespoons soy sauce (low sodium)

1 tablespoon rice vinegar

1 teaspoon grated ginger

1/4 teaspoon red pepper flakes (optional)

2 green onions, chopped

Sesame seeds for garnish

Instructions:


Cook lentils according to package instructions until tender. Drain and set aside.

In a large skillet or wok, heat olive oil over medium-high heat. Add onion and garlic, and sauté until fragrant.

Add bell pepper, zucchini, carrot, and broccoli. Stir-fry for 5-7 minutes, or until the vegetables are tender-crisp.

Add cooked lentils, soy sauce, rice vinegar, ginger, and red pepper flakes (if using). Stir well to combine.

Cook for an additional 2-3 minutes, allowing the flavors to meld together.

Garnish with green onions and sesame seeds. Serve over brown rice or quinoa.

## Side Dishes and Accompaniments

## Cauliflower Rice

Ingredients:

1 large head of cauliflower, chopped into florets

1 tablespoon olive oil

1 small onion, finely chopped

2 cloves garlic, minced

Salt and pepper to taste

Fresh parsley for garnish

Instructions:

Place cauliflower florets in a food processor and pulse until they resemble rice grains.

In a large skillet, heat olive oil over medium heat. Add onion and garlic, and sauté until translucent.

Add the cauliflower rice to the skillet and cook for 5-7 minutes, stirring occasionally, until tender.

Season with salt and pepper. Garnish with fresh parsley and serve as a low-carb side dish.

## Garlic Green Beans

Ingredients:

1 pound green beans, trimmed

2 tablespoons olive oil

4 cloves garlic, minced

Salt and pepper to taste

Lemon wedges for serving

Instructions:

Bring a large pot of water to a boil. Add the green beans and blanch for 3-4 minutes. Drain and set aside.

In a large skillet, heat olive oil over medium-high heat. Add garlic and sauté until golden.

Add the blanched green beans to the skillet. Cook for 5-7 minutes, stirring frequently, until tender.

Season with salt and pepper. Serve with lemon wedges for a zesty finish.

# Chapter 5.4: Snack and Dessert Recipes

Managing diabetes doesn't mean you have to give up delicious snacks and desserts. With thoughtful ingredient choices and mindful portion control, you can enjoy a variety of treats that won't spike your blood sugar levels. In this chapter, we'll explore a range of healthy, diabetes-friendly snacks and desserts that are both satisfying and easy to prepare.

Healthy Snacks for Diabetics

1. Greek Yogurt with Berries

Ingredients:

1 cup plain Greek yogurt

1/2 cup fresh berries (strawberries, blueberries, or raspberries)

1 tablespoon chia seeds

1 teaspoon honey (optional)

Instructions:

Spoon the Greek yogurt into a bowl.

Top with fresh berries and sprinkle with chia seeds.

Drizzle honey over the top if desired.

Serve immediately.

Benefits:

Greek yogurt is high in protein and probiotics, which can help stabilize blood sugar levels. Berries are low in sugar and high in fiber and antioxidants, making this snack both delicious and nutritious.

2. Veggie Sticks with Hummus

Ingredients:

1 cup baby carrots

1 cup cucumber slices

1 cup bell pepper strips

1/2 cup hummus

Instructions:

Arrange the vegetable sticks on a plate.

Serve with a bowl of hummus for dipping.

Benefits:

Vegetables are low in carbohydrates and rich in vitamins and minerals. Hummus, made from chickpeas, provides protein and healthy fats, making this a balanced and satisfying snack.

3. Apple Slices with Almond Butter

Ingredients:

1 medium apple, sliced

2 tablespoons almond butter

1 teaspoon cinnamon (optional)

Instructions:

Slice the apple into thin wedges.

Spread almond butter on each apple slice.

Sprinkle with cinnamon if desired.

Benefits:

Apples are high in fiber and water, helping to keep you full without raising blood sugar levels too quickly. Almond butter adds healthy fats and protein, which help to slow down the absorption of sugar.

## 4. Mixed Nuts and Seeds

Ingredients:

1/4 cup almonds

1/4 cup walnuts

1/4 cup pumpkin seeds

1/4 cup sunflower seeds

Instructions:

Mix all the nuts and seeds together in a bowl.

Store in an airtight container for a quick, on-the-go snack.

Benefits:

Nuts and seeds are packed with healthy fats, protein, and fiber. They are low in carbohydrates, making them an ideal snack for diabetics.

## Guilt-Free Desserts

### 1. Chia Pudding

Ingredients:

1/4 cup chia seeds

1 cup unsweetened almond milk

1 teaspoon vanilla extract

1 tablespoon maple syrup (optional)

Fresh berries for topping

Instructions:

In a bowl, combine chia seeds, almond milk, vanilla extract, and maple syrup.

Stir well and let it sit for 5 minutes. Stir again to prevent clumping.

Cover and refrigerate for at least 2 hours or overnight.

Top with fresh berries before serving.

Benefits:

Chia seeds are rich in omega-3 fatty acids, fiber, and protein. This pudding is low in carbohydrates and provides a slow release of energy, making it a great dessert option.

2. Avocado Chocolate Mousse

Ingredients:

2 ripe avocados

1/4 cup unsweetened cocoa powder

1/4 cup almond milk

2 tablespoons honey or maple syrup

1 teaspoon vanilla extract

Instructions:

Scoop the avocado flesh into a blender or food processor.

Add cocoa powder, almond milk, honey or maple syrup, and vanilla extract.

Blend until smooth and creamy.

Serve immediately or chill in the refrigerator before serving.

Benefits:

Avocados are high in healthy fats and fiber, which can help maintain stable blood sugar levels. This mousse is creamy and satisfying without the need for added sugars or unhealthy fats.

## 3. Baked Cinnamon Apples

Ingredients:

4 medium apples

1 tablespoon cinnamon

2 tablespoons water

1 tablespoon lemon juice

Instructions:

Preheat the oven to 350°F (175°C).

Core the apples and cut them into thin slices.

Place the apple slices in a baking dish and sprinkle with cinnamon.

Add water and lemon juice to the dish.

Bake for 20-25 minutes or until the apples are tender.

Serve warm or chilled.

Benefits:

Baked apples are a comforting dessert that provides fiber and natural sweetness without the need for added sugars. Cinnamon can help improve insulin sensitivity and lower blood sugar levels.

4. Coconut Flour Cookies

Ingredients:

1/2 cup coconut flour

1/4 cup coconut oil, melted

1/4 cup honey or maple syrup

2 eggs

1 teaspoon vanilla extract

1/4 teaspoon baking soda

A pinch of salt

Instructions:

Preheat the oven to 350°F (175°C) and line a baking sheet with parchment paper.

In a bowl, mix coconut flour, baking soda, and salt.

In another bowl, whisk together melted coconut oil, honey or maple syrup, eggs, and vanilla extract.

Combine the wet and dry ingredients and mix until a dough forms.

Scoop tablespoons of dough onto the baking sheet and flatten slightly.

Bake for 12-15 minutes or until the edges are golden brown.

Let cool before serving.

Benefits:

Coconut flour is low in carbohydrates and high in fiber, making it a great alternative to traditional flour for diabetics. These cookies are sweetened naturally and provide a satisfying treat without spiking blood sugar levels.

# 5.5: Beverage Recipes

In this section, we explore a variety of delicious and diabetes-friendly beverages that can be enjoyed throughout the year. These recipes include herbal teas, smoothies, juices, and low-sugar mocktails, all designed to help manage blood sugar levels while satisfying your taste buds. The following recipes are easy to prepare and include ingredients that can be readily found in most grocery stores.

## 1. Herbal Teas and Infusions

Herbal teas are a great way to enjoy the benefits of herbs while staying hydrated. Here are a few recipes that incorporate herbs known for their potential to help manage diabetes.

# Cinnamon and Ginger Tea

Ingredients:

1 cinnamon stick

1-inch piece of fresh ginger, sliced

2 cups of water

Optional: a slice of lemon, a few drops of stevia for sweetness

Instructions:

In a small pot, bring 2 cups of water to a boil.

Add the cinnamon stick and ginger slices to the boiling water.

Reduce the heat and let it simmer for 10 minutes.

Remove from heat and strain the tea into a cup.

Add a slice of lemon and a few drops of stevia if desired.

Enjoy warm or cold.

Benefits:

Cinnamon can help improve insulin sensitivity and lower blood sugar levels, while ginger has anti-inflammatory properties and can aid in digestion.

# Fenugreek and Mint Tea

Ingredients:

1 tablespoon fenugreek seeds

A handful of fresh mint leaves

2 cups of water

Optional: honey or stevia for sweetness

Instructions:

Soak the fenugreek seeds in 2 cups of water overnight.

In the morning, bring the fenugreek water to a boil along with the seeds.

Add the fresh mint leaves and let it simmer for 5 minutes.

Strain the tea into a cup.

Sweeten with honey or stevia if desired.

Enjoy warm or cold.

Benefits:

Fenugreek seeds have been shown to improve blood sugar control, and mint can aid in digestion and provide a refreshing flavor.

## 2. Smoothies and Juices

Smoothies and juices can be a nutritious way to incorporate fruits and vegetables into your diet. Here are some recipes that are low in sugar and high in fiber, making them suitable for diabetics.

Berry and Spinach Smoothie

Ingredients:

1 cup of fresh or frozen berries (strawberries, blueberries, raspberries)

1 cup of fresh spinach leaves

1/2 cup of plain Greek yogurt

1 cup of unsweetened almond milk

1 tablespoon chia seeds

Optional: a few drops of stevia for sweetness

Instructions:

Combine all ingredients in a blender.

Blend until smooth.

Pour into a glass and enjoy immediately.

Benefits:

Berries are low in sugar and high in antioxidants, while spinach provides essential vitamins and minerals. Chia seeds add fiber and omega-3 fatty acids.

Green Apple and Celery Juice

Ingredients:

1 green apple, cored and chopped

2 stalks of celery, chopped

1/2 cucumber, chopped

1-inch piece of fresh ginger, peeled and chopped

1/2 lemon, juiced

1 cup of water

Instructions:

Combine all ingredients in a blender.

Blend until smooth.

Strain the mixture through a fine mesh sieve or cheesecloth to remove the pulp.

Pour the juice into a glass and enjoy immediately.

Benefits:

Green apples are lower in sugar compared to other varieties, and celery is low in calories and high in fiber. Ginger adds a zesty flavor and aids in digestion.

## 3. Low-Sugar Mocktails

Mocktails are non-alcoholic beverages that can be enjoyed by everyone. Here are some refreshing options that are low in sugar and perfect for any occasion.

# Cucumber and Mint Cooler

Ingredients:

1 cucumber, thinly sliced

A handful of fresh mint leaves

1 tablespoon lime juice

1 tablespoon stevia or a low-calorie sweetener

4 cups of sparkling water

Ice cubes

Instructions:

In a pitcher, combine the cucumber slices, mint leaves, lime juice, and stevia.

Add ice cubes to the pitcher.

Pour the sparkling water over the ingredients.

Stir gently to combine.

Serve in glasses garnished with extra cucumber slices and mint leaves.

Benefits:

Cucumber is hydrating and low in calories, while mint adds a refreshing flavor without adding sugar. Lime juice provides a tangy taste and vitamin C.

# Berry Basil Lemonade

Ingredients:

1 cup of mixed berries (strawberries, blueberries, raspberries)

A handful of fresh basil leaves

1/2 cup of freshly squeezed lemon juice

1/4 cup stevia or a low-calorie sweetener

4 cups of water

Ice cubes

Instructions:

In a blender, combine the berries and basil leaves.

Blend until smooth.

Strain the berry-basil mixture through a fine mesh sieve to remove the pulp.

In a pitcher, combine the strained berry-basil juice, lemon juice, stevia, and water.

Stir well to combine.

Add ice cubes to the pitcher.

Serve in glasses garnished with extra basil leaves and berries.

Benefits:

Berries provide antioxidants and vitamins, while basil adds a unique flavor and potential anti-inflammatory benefits. Lemon juice is a good source of vitamin C and adds a refreshing tang.

# Chapter 6: Lifestyle Changes and Diabetes Management

## 6.1 The Importance of Exercise

Managing diabetes effectively requires more than just a careful diet and medication. Incorporating regular physical activity into daily life is a critical component of diabetes management. Exercise helps to regulate blood sugar levels, improves cardiovascular health, and enhances overall well-being. This section will explore the numerous benefits of exercise for individuals with diabetes, provide recommendations for various types of physical activities, and offer practical tips for integrating exercise into daily routines.

## Benefits of Physical Activity for Diabetics

Blood Sugar Regulation:

One of the most significant benefits of exercise for diabetics is its ability to help regulate blood sugar levels. When you engage in physical activity, your muscles use glucose for energy, which helps lower blood sugar levels. Additionally, exercise increases insulin sensitivity, meaning your cells can use available insulin more effectively to absorb glucose from the bloodstream. This dual action of reducing blood sugar and improving insulin sensitivity can significantly aid in managing diabetes.

Weight Management:

Maintaining a healthy weight is crucial for managing type 2 diabetes, and regular exercise is a key component of weight management. Physical activity burns calories, which helps in reducing body fat. Moreover, exercise can help build and maintain muscle mass, which further boosts metabolism and aids in weight control.

Cardiovascular Health:

Diabetics are at a higher risk of developing cardiovascular diseases. Regular exercise strengthens the heart and improves circulation, reducing the risk of heart attacks and strokes. It helps lower blood pressure, improves cholesterol levels by increasing HDL (good cholesterol) and decreasing LDL (bad cholesterol), and reduces triglycerides.

Mental Health Benefits:

Exercise has profound effects on mental health. It can help reduce stress, anxiety, and depression, all of which are common among individuals with diabetes. Physical activity promotes the release of endorphins, the body's natural mood lifters, leading to improved mood and emotional well-being. Regular exercise also enhances cognitive function and can improve sleep quality, contributing to overall mental health.

Improved Mobility and Joint Health:

Exercise, particularly strength training and flexibility exercises, can improve joint health and mobility. This is especially important for individuals with diabetes, who may be prone to joint issues and complications such as neuropathy. Improved joint health can enhance quality of life and enable greater independence in daily activities.

## Types of Exercise for Diabetics

Aerobic Exercise:

Aerobic exercises are activities that increase your heart rate and make you breathe harder. They are highly effective for improving cardiovascular health and aiding in weight management. Examples of aerobic exercises include:

Walking: A low-impact, accessible activity suitable for all fitness levels. Aim for at least 30 minutes of brisk walking most days of the week.

Running or Jogging: Higher intensity options for those who are more physically fit.

Cycling: Whether on a stationary bike or outdoors, cycling is an excellent cardiovascular workout.

Swimming: Provides a full-body workout and is gentle on the joints, making it ideal for individuals with arthritis or joint pain.

Dancing: A fun way to get your heart pumping while improving coordination and balance.

Strength Training:

Strength training involves exercises that build muscle mass and increase strength. It is essential for maintaining muscle mass, especially as we age, and for improving insulin sensitivity. Examples of strength training exercises include:

Weightlifting: Using free weights or weight machines to perform exercises like squats, deadlifts, and bench presses.

Bodyweight Exercises: Exercises such as push-ups, pull-ups, and squats that use your body weight for resistance.

Resistance Bands: Using elastic bands to provide resistance during exercises like bicep curls and leg presses.

Flexibility and Balance Exercises:

These exercises improve flexibility, reduce the risk of injury, and enhance balance and coordination. They are particularly beneficial for older adults and those with mobility issues. Examples include:

Stretching: Regular stretching routines can improve flexibility and range of motion.

Yoga: Combines flexibility, strength, and balance training, along with relaxation techniques.

Tai Chi: A gentle form of martial arts that improves balance, flexibility, and mental relaxation.

## Exercise Recommendations for Diabetics

Consult Your Healthcare Provider:

Before starting any exercise program, it's important to consult with your healthcare provider. They can help you design a safe and effective exercise plan tailored to your specific needs and medical condition.

Start Slowly:

If you are new to exercise or haven't been active for a while, start slowly and gradually increase the intensity and duration of your workouts. This approach helps prevent injury and makes it easier to stick with the program.

Set Realistic Goals:

Set achievable goals that are specific, measurable, attainable, relevant, and time-bound (SMART goals). For example, aim to walk for 20 minutes three times a week and gradually increase the duration and frequency.

## Monitor Blood Sugar Levels:

Keep track of your blood sugar levels before, during, and after exercise, especially if you are on insulin or other medications that can cause hypoglycemia (low blood sugar). Knowing how your body responds to different types of exercise can help you make necessary adjustments.

## Stay Hydrated:

Drink plenty of water before, during, and after exercise to stay hydrated. Dehydration can affect blood sugar levels and overall performance.

## Listen to Your Body:

Pay attention to how you feel during and after exercise. If you experience any unusual symptoms such as dizziness, shortness of breath, chest pain, or extreme fatigue, stop exercising and seek medical advice.

## Incorporate Variety:

Mix different types of exercises to keep your routine interesting and to work different muscle groups. This variety can prevent boredom and improve overall fitness.

## Find a Workout Buddy:

Exercising with a friend or joining a group class can provide motivation, accountability, and social interaction. A workout buddy can also offer support and encouragement.

Practical Tips for Integrating Exercise into Daily Routine

Schedule Exercise:

Treat exercise as an important appointment. Schedule it into your daily routine just like any other essential task.

Make it Enjoyable:

Choose activities that you enjoy. Whether it's dancing, hiking, or playing a sport, enjoying your workout increases the likelihood of sticking with it.

Use Technology:

Use fitness trackers, apps, and online resources to monitor your progress, set goals, and find new workouts. Many apps offer guided workouts and tips for staying active.

Incorporate Activity Throughout the Day:

Look for opportunities to be active throughout the day. Take the stairs instead of the elevator, walk or bike to work, or take short activity breaks during your workday.

Join a Class or Group:

Joining a fitness class or group can provide structure, variety, and social interaction. Many community centers, gyms, and online platforms offer classes tailored for different fitness levels and interests.

Be Consistent:

Consistency is key to reaping the benefits of exercise. Aim for at least 150 minutes of moderate-intensity aerobic activity or 75 minutes of vigorous-intensity activity each week, along with muscle-strengthening activities on two or more days a week.

# Chapter 6.2: Stress Management and Mental Health

Diabetes management is not just about controlling blood sugar levels through diet and medication; it also involves addressing the mental and emotional aspects of living with a chronic condition. Stress, in particular, can have a significant impact on blood sugar levels and overall health. In this section, we will explore the connection between stress and diabetes, the effects of chronic stress on mental health, and practical techniques for reducing stress and enhancing well-being.

## The Connection Between Stress and Blood Sugar

Stress is the body's natural response to challenging or threatening situations. When you experience stress, your body releases hormones like adrenaline and cortisol, which prepare you to react quickly—commonly known as the "fight or flight" response. While this response can be beneficial in short bursts, chronic stress can lead to sustained high levels of these hormones, which can adversely affect your health.

For individuals with diabetes, chronic stress can lead to:

Increased Blood Sugar Levels: Stress hormones like cortisol can cause the liver to release more glucose into the bloodstream, leading to elevated blood sugar levels. This can make it harder to manage diabetes effectively.

Insulin Resistance: Prolonged exposure to stress hormones can lead to insulin resistance, where the body's cells become less responsive to insulin. This can further complicate blood sugar management.

Poor Lifestyle Choices: Stress can influence behaviors and lifestyle choices that negatively impact diabetes management. For example, stressed individuals might turn to unhealthy comfort foods, skip exercise, or neglect their medication regimen.

## Effects of Chronic Stress on Mental Health

Living with diabetes can be stressful in itself, and the added burden of managing blood sugar levels, dietary restrictions, and potential complications can take a toll on mental health. Chronic stress can lead to a range of mental health issues, including:

Anxiety: Persistent worry about blood sugar levels, potential complications, and the future can cause anxiety. This can manifest as physical symptoms like increased heart rate, sweating, and difficulty sleeping.

Depression: The constant pressure of managing a chronic condition can lead to feelings of hopelessness, sadness, and a lack of interest in activities once enjoyed. Depression can also negatively impact diabetes management, creating a vicious cycle.

Burnout: Diabetes burnout occurs when individuals feel overwhelmed by the daily demands of diabetes management. This can lead to neglecting important aspects of care, such as monitoring blood sugar levels and adhering to a healthy diet.

Techniques for Reducing Stress

Managing stress is crucial for overall well-being and effective diabetes management. Here are several practical techniques that can help reduce stress and improve mental health:

Mindfulness and Meditation:

Mindfulness: Practicing mindfulness involves focusing on the present moment without judgment. This can help reduce anxiety and improve emotional regulation. Techniques include deep breathing exercises, mindful eating, and guided imagery.

Meditation: Regular meditation can lower stress hormone levels and promote relaxation. Even a few minutes of daily meditation can have significant benefits.

Physical Activity:

Exercise is a natural stress reliever. Physical activity helps release endorphins, which are chemicals in the brain that act as natural painkillers and mood elevators. Activities like walking, yoga, swimming, and dancing can be effective in reducing stress.

Social Support:

Building a strong support network is vital. Talking to friends, family, or support groups about your feelings and experiences can provide emotional relief and practical advice. Support groups, both online and in-person, offer a sense of community and understanding.

Healthy Lifestyle Choices:

Nutrition: Eating a balanced diet can help stabilize mood and energy levels. Avoid excessive caffeine and sugar, which can contribute to anxiety and mood swings.

Sleep: Adequate sleep is essential for mental health. Establishing a regular sleep routine and creating a restful environment can improve sleep quality.

Professional Help:

Seeking help from mental health professionals, such as psychologists or counselors, can provide valuable coping strategies and therapeutic interventions. Cognitive-behavioral therapy (CBT) is particularly effective for managing anxiety and depression.

Time Management:

Organizing your day and prioritizing tasks can reduce feelings of overwhelm. Breaking tasks into smaller, manageable steps and setting realistic goals can help you feel more in control.

Relaxation Techniques:

Activities such as listening to music, reading, spending time in nature, and engaging in hobbies can provide relaxation and a mental break from daily stresses.

Integrating Stress Management into Daily Life

To effectively manage stress and improve mental health, it is essential to incorporate these techniques into your daily routine. Here are some tips for making stress management a regular part of your life:

Set Aside Time for Self-Care: Dedicate a specific time each day for activities that promote relaxation and well-being.

Be Consistent: Regular practice of stress management techniques can lead to lasting benefits. Consistency is key to making these practices a habit.

Monitor Your Progress: Keep a journal to track your stress levels and the effectiveness of different techniques. This can help you identify what works best for you.

Stay Positive: Focus on the positive aspects of your life and practice gratitude. This can shift your perspective and improve your overall outlook.

# 6.3 Monitoring Blood Sugar Levels

Monitoring blood sugar levels is a crucial component of diabetes management. It helps individuals with diabetes understand how their diet, physical activity, medications, and other lifestyle factors impact their blood glucose levels. Effective monitoring can prevent complications, improve overall health, and enable individuals to take proactive steps in managing their condition. This section will cover the importance of monitoring, how to use a glucometer, understanding blood sugar readings, and best practices for effective monitoring.

## The Importance of Monitoring Blood Sugar Levels

For individuals with diabetes, keeping blood sugar levels within a target range is essential. Consistently high blood sugar levels can lead to complications such as heart disease, kidney damage, nerve damage, and vision problems. Conversely, low blood sugar levels (hypoglycemia) can cause symptoms like dizziness, confusion, and even loss of consciousness. Monitoring blood sugar levels regularly helps in:

Preventing Complications: By identifying and addressing high or low blood sugar levels promptly, individuals can avoid severe complications.

Adjusting Treatment Plans: Regular monitoring provides data that can help healthcare providers adjust medications, dietary plans, and physical activity levels to better manage diabetes.

Empowering Individuals: Monitoring allows individuals to understand their body's response to various foods, activities, and medications, empowering them to make informed decisions about their health.

Improving Quality of Life: Effective blood sugar management can lead to improved energy levels, better mood, and overall enhanced quality of life.

## How to Use a Glucometer

A glucometer is a small, portable device used to measure blood glucose levels. Here are the steps to use a glucometer:

Wash Your Hands: Ensure your hands are clean to avoid contamination. Use warm water to improve blood flow if necessary.

Prepare the Device: Insert a test strip into the glucometer. Ensure the device is calibrated if needed.

Lance Your Finger: Use a lancet to prick the side of your fingertip. This is less painful than pricking the pad of your finger.

Obtain a Blood Sample: Gently squeeze your finger to obtain a drop of blood. Place the drop on the test strip.

Read the Results: The glucometer will display your blood glucose level on the screen within a few seconds.

Record the Results: Keep a log of your readings, including the date, time, and any relevant notes such as recent meals or activities.

Understanding Blood Sugar Readings

Blood sugar readings provide valuable insights into how well diabetes is being managed. Here's how to interpret the results:

Fasting Blood Sugar Levels: These readings are taken after at least 8 hours of fasting. The target range for fasting blood sugar is typically between 70 and 130 mg/dL.

Postprandial Blood Sugar Levels: These readings are taken 1-2 hours after a meal. The target range for postprandial blood sugar is usually less than 180 mg/dL.

Random Blood Sugar Levels: These readings can be taken at any time of the day, regardless of when you last ate. Target ranges may vary, but a random blood sugar level below 140 mg/dL is generally considered normal.

Interpreting the Results:

Within Target Range: If your blood sugar levels are within the target range, it indicates good diabetes management. Continue following your current treatment plan.

Above Target Range: High blood sugar levels (hyperglycemia) may indicate that your body isn't producing enough insulin or that your cells are resistant to insulin. Factors contributing to high readings could include excessive carbohydrate intake, insufficient medication, stress, or lack of physical activity. High blood sugar levels require adjustments in diet, medication, or lifestyle to prevent complications.

Below Target Range: Low blood sugar levels (hypoglycemia) can occur if you take too much insulin, skip meals, or engage in strenuous exercise without adjusting your food intake. Symptoms of hypoglycemia include sweating, shaking, confusion, and irritability. Immediate consumption of fast-acting carbohydrates (e.g., glucose tablets, fruit juice) can help raise blood sugar levels.

Best Practices for Effective Monitoring

To ensure accurate and effective blood sugar monitoring, consider the following best practices:

Regular Monitoring: Check your blood sugar levels at times recommended by your healthcare provider. This may include before meals, after meals, before and after exercise, and before bed.

Consistent Record Keeping: Maintain a detailed log of your blood sugar readings, noting the date, time, and any factors that might have influenced the results. Digital apps and glucose meters with memory functions can help streamline this process.

Responding to Readings: Use your blood sugar readings to make informed decisions about your diet, physical activity, and medication. For example, if your blood sugar is high after a meal, consider adjusting your portion sizes or carbohydrate intake for future meals.

Regular Calibration and Maintenance: Ensure your glucometer is functioning correctly by following the manufacturer's guidelines for calibration and maintenance. Replace the batteries as needed and store test strips in a cool, dry place.

Education and Support: Stay informed about diabetes management through education and support groups. Engaging with healthcare providers, diabetes educators, and support communities can provide valuable insights and encouragement.

Healthy Lifestyle Choices: Complement blood sugar monitoring with a healthy lifestyle. A balanced diet, regular physical activity, adequate sleep, and stress management all play a vital role in maintaining stable blood sugar levels.

# Chapter 6.4: Long-term Strategies for Success

Managing diabetes is a lifelong journey that requires dedication, consistency, and a proactive approach. While immediate dietary changes and exercise routines can have a significant impact on blood sugar levels, maintaining these improvements over the long term is crucial for sustained health benefits. In this section, we will explore effective strategies to help you set realistic goals, stay motivated, and remain consistent in your diabetes management efforts.

Setting Realistic Goals

One of the most important aspects of long-term diabetes management is setting realistic and achievable goals. Unrealistic expectations can lead to frustration and burnout, making it harder to stay on track. Here are some key considerations for setting effective goals:

Specific and Measurable: Goals should be specific and measurable. For example, instead of setting a vague goal like "eat healthier," aim for something more concrete like "include at least one serving of vegetables in every meal." This makes it easier to track progress and make adjustments as needed.

Attainable and Relevant: Ensure that your goals are attainable and relevant to your overall health objectives. Setting goals that are too ambitious can be discouraging. For instance, if you're not used to exercising regularly, start with a goal of walking for 10 minutes a day, then gradually increase the duration as you build endurance.

Time-bound: Goals should have a clear timeframe. Short-term goals can provide immediate motivation, while long-term goals help you stay focused on your overall health journey. For example, set a goal to reduce your HbA1c levels by a specific percentage within six months.

Flexible and Adaptable: Life is unpredictable, and it's important to be flexible with your goals. If you encounter setbacks, reassess and adjust your goals rather than giving up entirely. Flexibility helps you stay committed even when faced with challenges.

Staying Motivated

Maintaining motivation over the long term can be challenging, but it's essential for sustained success in diabetes management. Here are some strategies to keep your motivation levels high:

Celebrate Small Wins: Recognize and celebrate small achievements along the way. Whether it's successfully sticking to your meal plan for a week or completing a new exercise routine, acknowledging these victories can boost your confidence and motivation.

Track Your Progress: Keeping a record of your progress can provide a visual reminder of how far you've come. Use a journal, app, or chart to track your blood sugar levels, dietary habits, and physical activity. Seeing positive trends can reinforce your commitment.

Find Support: Connecting with others who are also managing diabetes can provide valuable support and encouragement. Join a support group, participate in online forums, or partner with a friend or family member to share experiences and stay motivated together.

Set New Challenges: Keep things interesting by setting new challenges for yourself. Trying new recipes, exploring different types of physical activities, or setting personal records can add variety and excitement to your routine.

Remember Your Why: Reflect on the reasons why you want to manage your diabetes effectively. Whether it's to improve your health, increase your energy levels, or be there for your loved ones, keeping your motivations in mind can help you stay focused.

Staying Consistent

Consistency is key to long-term success in diabetes management. Here are some tips to help you maintain consistency in your efforts:

Establish Routines: Creating daily routines can help make healthy habits a regular part of your life. Set specific times for meals, exercise, and medication to ensure you stay on track. Routines reduce decision fatigue and make it easier to stick to your plan.

Plan Ahead: Preparation is crucial for consistency. Plan your meals and snacks in advance, and keep healthy options readily available. Schedule regular exercise sessions and set reminders for medication and blood sugar monitoring.

Stay Educated: Keep yourself informed about diabetes management and stay updated on the latest research and recommendations. Knowledge empowers you to make informed decisions and adapt to changes as needed.

Adjust as Needed: Your body and circumstances may change over time, requiring adjustments to your management plan. Regularly review your goals and strategies, and consult with your healthcare team to make necessary modifications.

Practice Self-Compassion: Be kind to yourself and understand that perfection is not the goal. There will be times when you slip up or face challenges. Instead of being overly critical, practice self-compassion and focus on getting back on track.

Long-term Health Benefits

Sticking to these strategies not only helps manage diabetes but also contributes to overall health and well-being. Consistent blood sugar control can reduce the risk of complications such as cardiovascular disease, kidney damage, and neuropathy. Additionally, maintaining a healthy diet and regular physical activity can improve your energy levels, mental health, and quality of life.

By setting realistic goals, staying motivated, and maintaining consistency, you can effectively manage your diabetes and enjoy a healthier, more fulfilling life. Remember, the journey is ongoing, and every positive step you take brings you closer to long-term success in managing your diabetes.

# Chapter 7: Success Stories and Testimonials

## 7.1 Case Studies of Reversed Diabetes

Real-life Success Stories

One of the most compelling aspects of any health-related book is the inclusion of real-life success stories. These narratives not only inspire readers but also provide tangible evidence that the recommended approaches can work. In this section, we will delve into several case studies where individuals successfully managed or even reversed their diabetes through Dr. Barbara O'Neill's methods.

## Case Study 1: John's Journey to Health

John, a 45-year-old man diagnosed with type 2 diabetes, struggled with managing his blood sugar levels for years. Despite trying various medications and diets, his HbA1c levels remained stubbornly high. After discovering Dr. Barbara O'Neill's approach, John decided to overhaul his lifestyle. He adopted the 28-day meal plan and incorporated the recommended herbal remedies into his daily routine. Within three months, John's blood sugar levels stabilized, and his HbA1c dropped significantly. His energy levels increased, and he lost 20 pounds, transforming his life completely.

## Case Study 2: Mary's Path to Reversing Type 1 Diabetes

Mary, diagnosed with type 1 diabetes at the age of 12, believed she would be dependent on insulin for life. Upon learning about Dr. Barbara's methods, she was intrigued but skeptical. Mary decided to gradually integrate the herbal remedies and dietary changes into her regimen. Over time, she noticed a remarkable improvement in her blood sugar control. Though she still required insulin, her dosage reduced significantly, and her overall health improved. Mary's story highlights that while type 1 diabetes cannot be completely reversed, Dr. Barbara's methods can lead to substantial health benefits.

## Case Study 3: Linda's Success with Gestational Diabetes

Linda was diagnosed with gestational diabetes during her second pregnancy. Worried about the impact on her unborn child, she sought alternative approaches to manage her condition. By following Dr. Barbara's meal plans and using specific herbal remedies, Linda maintained stable blood sugar levels throughout her pregnancy. She delivered a healthy baby and successfully avoided the complications often associated with gestational diabetes.

Interviews with Successful Individuals

In addition to written testimonials, conducting interviews with individuals who have successfully managed their diabetes using Dr. Barbara's methods can provide deeper insights. These interviews can be formatted as Q&A sessions, offering readers a personal perspective on the challenges and triumphs faced by these individuals.

Interview with John

Q: What motivated you to try Dr. Barbara O'Neill's approach?

A: I was tired of feeling sick and tired all the time. Medications weren't giving me the results I wanted, and I was desperate for a change. When I read about Dr. Barbara's methods, I felt a glimmer of hope and decided to give it a shot.

Q: What was the most challenging part of the journey?

A: The initial transition was tough. Changing my eating habits and incorporating herbs I wasn't familiar with took some getting used to. But once I saw the positive changes in my health, it became easier to stick with it.

Q: How has your life changed since adopting this approach?

A: My energy levels are through the roof, and I feel better than I have in years. My blood sugar levels are stable, and I've lost a significant amount of weight. It's been a life-changing experience.

# 7.2 Testimonials from Dr. Barbara's Clients

Testimonials from Dr. Barbara's clients can offer readers relatable and encouraging stories of success. These personal accounts provide authenticity and reinforce the effectiveness of her methods. Here are a few examples:

# Client Testimonial 1: Sarah's Transformation

"I was diagnosed with type 2 diabetes five years ago and struggled to control my blood sugar levels. After attending one of Dr. Barbara's seminars, I decided to follow her recommendations. The 28-day meal plan was a game-changer for me. I learned how to prepare delicious, diabetes-friendly meals and incorporated the herbal remedies she suggested. Within months, my blood sugar levels were under control, and I felt healthier than ever. I'm grateful for Dr. Barbara's guidance and support."

# Client Testimonial 2: Mike's Journey to Better Health

"Being diagnosed with diabetes was a wake-up call for me. I knew I needed to make significant changes to my lifestyle. Dr. Barbara's approach was exactly what I needed. The combination of diet, herbal remedies, and lifestyle changes made a huge difference. My blood sugar levels are now within the normal range, and I've lost 30 pounds. Dr. Barbara's methods work, and I'm living proof of that."

## Lessons Learned from Dr. Barbara's Approach

These testimonials not only highlight success stories but also share valuable lessons learned along the way. Readers can gain insights into the practical aspects of adopting a new lifestyle and the perseverance required to achieve lasting results.

**Key Lesson 1: Consistency is Crucial**

One common theme among the testimonials is the importance of consistency. Adopting a new lifestyle and sticking with it can be challenging, but the benefits are well worth the effort. Clients emphasize that staying consistent with the meal plans and herbal remedies is key to seeing significant improvements in health.

**Key Lesson 2: Support Systems Matter**

Another important lesson is the value of having a support system. Many clients mentioned that having the support of family, friends, or a community of like-minded individuals helped them stay motivated and on track. Dr. Barbara's seminars and online communities provide a network of support for those embarking on this journey.

# 7.3 Additional Resources and Support

**Online Communities and Support Groups**

Joining online communities and support groups can be incredibly beneficial for individuals managing diabetes. These platforms offer a space for sharing experiences, asking questions, and receiving encouragement from others on a similar journey. Here are some recommended online resources:

**Dr. Barbara O'Neill's Online Community**: An online forum where individuals can share their experiences, ask questions, and receive support from Dr. Barbara and other members.

**Diabetes Support Groups:** Websites like Diabetes.co.uk and the American Diabetes Association offer forums and support groups for individuals living with diabetes.

**Social Media Groups:** Facebook and other social media platforms have numerous groups dedicated to diabetes management and support.

Made in the USA
Las Vegas, NV
12 July 2024

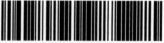

92230624R00107